The Healing
Essentials of Clay

Amanda Sarita Del Forte

authorHOUSE®

AuthorHouse™
1663 Liberty Drive, Suite 200
Bloomington, IN 47403
www.authorhouse.com
Phone: 1-800-839-8640

First published by AuthorHouse 3/12/2009

ISBN: 978-1-4389-4967-3 (sc)

Scripture references within this book are from the King
James version of *The Holy Bible*.

Printed in the United States of America
Bloomington, Indiana

This book is printed on acid-free paper.

This book is dedicated especially to my immediate family: My husband, Louis, Sons (Darwin) Danthony and Amy and Daughters Deborah and Dija as well as my grand-children, D. J.(Darwin Jr) Devian, Dominique, Demi and Joey, Jeremiah and Michael. (also to my extended family) Too many to mention, but you know who you are.

Most of all, I give all glory and Honor to my Lord Jesus Christ for His presence in my life. If you desire to be healthy the natural way, then this book is for you.

Disclaimer:

I am not a Medical Doctor or a veterinarian; and I am not advising you to perform any of these remedies without advice from a medical doctor. I personally know that there are many good medical doctors in our society, and I do visit them when the time requires me to do so. Remember also that Luke in the bible was a physician. *However, the remedies found in this book are personal benefits I have personally found to work for myself and others; and are to be used at your own discretion; Also, are listed personal testimonies of other individuals obtained from various other sources of research who have benefited by using clay therapy.*

The Healing Essentials of Clay

What is dirt? Dirt is made up of : (in the earths atmosphere for plant growth) **SOIL=PLANTS=LIFE**

Again , the answer is: No! dirt isn't just dirt....*It is Life!*....(Dirt mixed with a liquid=clay)

*Websters New Dictionary states dirt as: a Noun and is **Earth, or Mud.Dictionary.Com unabridged v1.1** cite the source of dirt is (a noun) and is earth, as mud or dust, soil, especially when loose.*

Listed below is a brief introduction into the contents of the basics of the earth minerals (natural clay components) as well as the elements in the human body...

The ones highlighted in bold print are the same essentials found in plants, (from soil) as well as found in the human body.

Oxygen	**46.5%**
Silicon	28.0%
Aluminum	8.1 %
Iron	**5.1 %**
Calcium	**3.5 %**
Sodium	**3.0 %**
Potassium	**2.5 %**
Magnesium	2.2 %
Titanium	0.5 %

Through geophysical forces, mixing of the earth's crust with water can provide virtually every mineral our body requires to maintain health. This explains why the noted nutritionists, **Ruth L. Pike and Myrtle L. Brown** stated in Nutrition: An integrated Approach(**John Wiley**

and Sons), 1984, p. 197) *that: water is compatible with more substances than any known solvent, and therefore it is an ideal medium for mammals.*

----each of us carries in our veins a salty stream in which the elements are combined in almost the same proportions as in sea water

"Sixteen elements are absolutely necessary for normal plant growth. Many of these elements are the same as those required by humans. In addition to carbon, hydrogen, and oxygen, which the plant gets from the air and water another , another thirteen elements are required by plants, which they obtain from the **soil.**

Minerals essential for the human body:

(Listed below in the ***bold highlight*** are the minerals found in the body as well as in the earth and plants)

Boron: assists, improves retention of calcium, magnesium, and phosphorus; necessary for brain function, memory and alertness as well as for the activation of vitamin D.

Calcium: found mainly in bones and teeth-important for membrane function, nerve impulses, muscle contractions, and blood clotting.

Not only important for strong bones and teeth, it is also needed for the nervous system, muscle growth and heart regulation. It prevents acid-alkaline imbalances in the blood. The best sources of calcium are dairy products and bone products (liquid calcium, etc.) Sufficient vitamin D is needed for calcium absorption as is a proper potassium / calcium ratio in the blood. An excess of sugar and mental stress can pull calcium from the bones.

Carbon: found in all organic molecules
The Best Sources of Carbon are:
1. Sugars (natural) sweet fruits: starches; grains; breads; fats; cheeses; most proteins; meats; fish
2. Avocados, apples dried pears
3. Almonds
4. Apricots
5. Butter, turkey
6. Cream
7. Egg yolk, rice, yellow cornmeal
8. Olive and peanut oils
9. Figs, grapes lentils wheat germ and bran

Chlorine: important for membrane function and water absorption; chloride is the major anion in body fluids and part of hydrochloric acid in gastric juices.

Chromium: master regulator of insulin; potent metabolic hormone in the metabolism of proteins, carbohydrates and fats. Helps with the function of the brain, thyroid and hormonal balance.

Cobalt: a vital part of vitamin B12: stimulates numerous enzymes; helps build red blood cells and with iron absorption.

Copper: involved in the synthesis of hemoglobin, melanin, and elastin;
The Best Sources of Copper are:
1. Calf's liver, braised
2. Sesame seeds
3. Cashews, raw
4. Crimini Mushrooms, raw
5. Soybeans, cooked

* Copper helps your body utilize iron
* Reduce tissue damage caused by free radicals
*Maintain healthy bones and connective tissues
* Help your body produce the pigment called
Melanin (skin)
* Keep your thyroid gland functioning normally
* Preserve the myelin sheath that surrounds and
protects your nerves

Indications for a more high-copper diet:
*Iron deficiency anemia
*Blood vessels that rupture easily
* Bone and Joint problems
* Elevated LDL cholesterol and reduced HDL
cholesterol levels
* Frequent infections
* Loss of Hair or skin color
* Fatigue and weakness
* Difficulty breathing and irregular heart beat
* Skin sores

Germanium: helps activate various organs to attract more oxygen; helps maintain a strong immune system.
Hydrogen: a component of water and most other compounds in the body.
Iodine: a major component of thyroid hormones necessary for the metabolism of fats and such minerals as calcium, silica, and phosphorus; essential for spleen, liver and brain function; neutralizes albumin.

Iron: essential for oxygen transport and energy capture. Iron is an essential for the formation of hemoglobin. The iron in hemoglobin combines with oxygen and transports it through the blood to all parts of the body. Anemia is a result of *iron deficiency*. As a result of anemia, the person has symptoms of tiredness, lack of stamina, headaches, insomnia, breathlessness, and loss of appetite. These symptoms or signs show an iron deficiency.

Vegetables like broccoli and bok choy (dark green vegetables) are rich in iron, and also high in vitamin C, which increases absorption of their iron content. The presence of vitamin C in these vegetables help absorb iron. The amount of iron absorbed from vegetarian foods is about 1-10%, while it is 10-20% from animal foods. Combinations such as beans and tomato or tofu and broccoli result in good iron absorption.

One cup of cooked spinach contains 3 mg, one cup of tofu contains 13.2 mg. and one cup cooked lentils give 6.4 mg of iron.

Top Ten Iron Rich Foods:
Clams, cooked (3 oz) (23.8 mg)
Tofu ½ cup firm (13.2 mg)
Raisin bran (¾ cup (4.5 mg.)
Sirloin steak, cooked 3 0z (2.9 mg)
Shrimp, cooked 3 oz. (2.6 mg)
Black beans, boiled, ½ cup (1.8 mg.)
Chickpeas, canned ,½ cup (1.6 mg)
Turkey breast, 3 oz. (0.9 mg)
Bread, whole wheat 1 slice (0.9 mg.)
Chicken breast, skinless, ½ breast (0.9 mg)

<u>Magnesium:</u> Vital function, calms nerves; promotes

cell growth.

This mineral is essential for enzyme activity, calcium and potassium uptake, the formation of bone structure and metabolism of carbohydrates and minerals. High levels in water for consumption for the human body have found to be high in the resistance to heart disease.

Sources of magnesium are:
1. Dairy Products
2. Nuts
3. Vegetables
4. Fish
5. Meat
6. Seafood

Magnesium deficiency can result in coronary heart disease , obesity, fatigue, impaired brain functions. It has been said that chocolate cravings are a sign of magnesium deficiency.

Manganese: strengthens nerves and thought processes; helps with eyesight; helps with body's recuperative abilities and resistance to disease.

Nitrogen: found in proteins (78% of the air we breathe is nitrogen but only 21%

Nitrogen sources found in:
1. High protein foods
2. Nuts
3. Fish
4. Pasta
5. Cheeses

6. Ripe olives

<u>Nitrogen </u>is the "restrainer" element.
It vitalizes, builds tissues and is found in the body tissues, elastic and connective tissue, hair and nails, skin, lens of eye; is essential for complete metabolism.

Nitrogen in conjunction with the other three vital elements (hydrogen, oxygen and carbon) is important for life, power and vigor in all organisms. In order for metabolism to be complete nitrogen is essential in all forms:

<u>Oxygen</u>: a component of water and other compounds. Oxygen gas is essential for respiration.

Best sources of oxygen in foods are:

***<u>Fresh vegetables and fruits eaten without cooking</u>:

.<u>Phosphorus</u>: found in the nucleus of every cell in the body and is necessary for the reproductive system and sexual function, necessary for muscle tissue and growth, an essential nutrient for the nerves.

Phosphorus is an essential mineral that is usually found in nature combined with oxygen as phosphate. Most of the phosphate in the human body is bone, but phosphate-containing molecules are also important components of cell membranes and lipoprotein particles, such as HDL and LDL (good and bad cholesterols. Small amounts of phosphate play important roles in numerous biochemical reactions throughout the body.

Phosphorus is found in most foods because it is a critical component of all living organisms. Dairy products, meat, and fish are particularly rich sources of phosphorus. ** <u>Phosphorus is also a component of many polyphosphate food additives and is present in most soft drinks as phosphoric acid.</u>

Sources of Phosphates:

1. Protein rich foods
2. Cereal grains
3. Approximately 85% of the body's phosphorus is found in bone.
4. Beans, peas, nuts

<u>(for more information on the nutrient content of foods, search the USDA food composition database.)</u>
<u>Jane Higdon, PhD Linus Pauling Institute</u>
<u>Oregon State University (April, 2003)</u>
<u>Victoria J. Drake, Ph.D.</u>
<u>Linus Pauling Institute</u>
<u>Oregon State University</u>
<u>James P. Knochel, M.D.</u>
<u>Clinical Professor, Emeritus Presbyterian Hospital</u>
<u>University of Texas Southwestern Medical School</u>

<u>Potassium:</u> important for proper membrane function, nerve impulses, and muscle contraction; helps eliminate toxins from the body.

It is an element (and an electrolyte) that's essential for the body's growth and maintenance.

Potassium and sodium work together...The inner cell fluids are high in potassium while on the other hand while the fluids outside the cell are high in sodium. Therefore, potassium is important for many chemical reactions within the cells. It is also important in treating high blood pressure.(hypertension)

Sources of potassium are:

1. Bananas
2. Cantaloupes
3. Grapefruit
4. Oranges
5. Tomato or prune juice
6. Molasses
7. Potatoes

Note:

Excessive use of salt along with inadequate intake of fruits and vegetables can result in a potassium deficiency.

Selenium: a powerful antioxidant; vital to the immune system; supports heart function, helps maintain cell integrity.

Sodium: stored in stomach walls, joints and gallbladder; helps prevent blood clotting; important for membrane function; works with the bicarbonate buffer system in the digestive system to prevent hydrochloric acid from burning stomach walls.

Sulphur: increases blood circulation, reduces muscle cramping, regulates heart and brain function; promotes healthy skin, nails and hair; helps lubricate joints.

Zinc: found in all body fluids, including urine as well as the moisture found in the eyes, mouth, lungs and nose; necessary for normal taste sensation, wound healing, and a vital part of the immune system.

****We have seen that the minerals listed below

**are found in the soil as well as in our human body.
(the minerals below that are in bold type)
Oxygen:
Iron:
Calcium:
Sodium:
Potassium:
Phosphorus:**

Now that you've found out that some of the elements found in plants as well as the comparison to the human body, we can began looking at some practical applications. (their usages and where they are found)

Minerals are present in living tissue and are essential to all chemical reactions in the body. However, the body cannot manufacture its own minerals, and they must therefore be supplied by an outside source. Without minerals, the body will easily succumb to disease.

What do minerals do?

Supply major elements and trace elements that may be lacking in the diet.

Act as a catalyst, thus playing a major role in metabolism and cell building.

Regulate the permeability of cell membrane.

Maintain water balance and osmotic pressure between the inside and outside environment.

Influences the contractility of muscles.

Regulate the response of nerves to stimuli.

In this book, I discuss the beneficial healing properties of clay as well as other natural healing methods in maintaining a healthy lifestyle.

I began looking the properties in dirt, mixed with

a liquid =(clay) in 1985 when I took a class in Chinese medicine____an elective I chose for my continuing education requirements for my nursing license renewal.

During the class someone brought up the topic of survival without food.....At that point I thought of dirt (or clay, mixed with water or liquid)....Everything we consume is basically formed naturally in the soil. The vegetables we eat comes from the soil.....the animals we eat...consumes grasses and grains from the earth...

Everywhere you look, everyone is talking about natural ideas and medicines, and natural hormones.

Why hasn't clay (dirt) the source of all the natural medicine become the focal point of discussion?.--After all, that is in actuality, *our beginning....*

Scripture reference, KJV:

These are the generations of the heavens and of the earth when they were created, in the day that the Lord God made the earth and the heavens,

5 And every plant of the field before it was in the earth, and every herb of the field before it grew: for the Lord God had not caused it to rain upon the earth, and *there was* not a man to till the ground.

6 But there went up a mist from the earth, and watered the whole face of the earth, and watered the whole face of the ground.

7 And the Lord God formed man of the dust of the ground and breathed into his nostrils the breath of life; and man became a living soul.

8 And the Lord God planted a garden eastward in Eden; and there he put the man whom he had formed.

9 And out of the ground made the Lord God to grow

every tree that is pleasant to the sight, and good for food;...Genesis 2:4-9

The main reason for the publication of this book is to share with others what I have learned personally <u>about the healing properties of clay.</u> Everyone has faith in some type of healing processes, whether natural or from *some other source...*

There is a time however, when it is vital for you to seek help from a medical doctor, and there are other times also when you can use the natural healing processes that are right in front of you: and these processes are natural, from the earth.

In recent years, clay has been thought of in a different light, or perhaps an idea? Or a "possibility".

On march 19,1997, a T.V. show "extra" magazine did broadcast a five minute feature on clay....actually the eating of clay, a major plug for geophagy, and some time ago PBS aired an hour special <u>on geophagy</u>(the eating of clay) pronounced (gee-off-uh-gee), **Ran Knishinsky**. Unfortunately, our earth as God has created it, discusts many. Uniformed individuals, to the point of them calling dirt "dirty and unclean". However, they will consume foods that they knowingly contain pesticides and various poisons. They even feed these foods to their children. They will even shower and drink water that is filled with chlorine, and will breathe in cancerous fumes and vapors from factories and dyes.....but they will not even "consider" the life giving properties of "dirt or clay".

Although clay is not a miracle cure for all disease, I personally have found it beneficial in many instances. **Again, it is not a *quick cure* for any medical problem.**

It has a great deal to do with your personal habits on a daily basis.

How much do you want relief from the situation? Especially if it is a serious one.

Are you willing to do what is necessary to rid yourself of the problem?

(For instance, are you a chain-smoker? Are you a violent, angry individual? Do you consume fast foods every day? There are many other habits that create an unhealthy lifestyle. If you keep these habits and practice them daily, it will be a matter of time until they will catch up to you, and illnesses will begin to emerge. At this time you have to make a decision whether to *stop immediately* or …resume.

I'm sure you realize what the ultimate results will be.)

Healing clay also acts on behalf on all the organs. Everything that emits negative radiations (*everything unhealthy*) is attracted to clay and becomes subject to elimination. It is a very effective detoxifier.

And as all medicines and cures, one should use **Godly wisdom.** Do you question your doctor about the medicines you put into your body? How beneficial are they to you? If you take them over a certain amount of time, how will they effect your body?

However, personally I would not use clay that has been exposed to **known** toxins, such as inner city clay where there is an influx of people and pollution. Also a commercial farm area where pesticides are infused into the soil. As I have stated before, one should use **Godly wisdom** and be selective. However, you can, if you want it enough_find the right clay for your specific purpose; which is God's wonderful creation of life!

17

I found that when an individuals mind is open and can receive constructive information concerning a healing method and will use the information to their own need, it will work for them; but they have to have faith for it... the same as if they have faith for a medication the doctor prescribes. The mud therapy procedures work great also if your mind is tuned directly to God and you can first undergo a cleansing fast of fruits and vegetables. Your mind has a great deal to do with the success of your healing in certain instances. A negative or positive reaction. **Remember, you say what you get!!!!**

Remember, God gave to us Divine as well as natural healing.

Scripture: Proverbs 18:21 The power of life and death is in your tongue: and they that love it shall eat the fruit thereof....

..To get a positive result from the treatment, you must keep an open and receiving mind. You will even get some results with an unbelieving mind. To get maximum results, it helps to have a relaxed receiving attitude and confess healing scriptures daily..

I remembered the passage in the bible where Jesus applied mud to the eyes of the blind man. *(John 9:1-11)* Also I remember when Jesus told the man with leprosy to dip himself seven times in the muddy Jordan river (*2 Kings 5:1-14)*

A few years ago, my daughter, Debbie developed a cyst on her coccyx area(her lower back) She had it previously lanced by a medical doctor, but it did re-occur awhile later. During this time she was having difficulty walking.

She called me and at that time, I made a bed for her in

Turmeric & Clay . . .

the bath-tub, and there I applied the mud directly on the cyst. It was a combination of mud and tumeric spice.(an anti inflammatory) She told me that she remained on her abdomen for a few hours. Later, she showered and went to bed. She stated that later when she used the bathroom, she felt something warm running down her lower back. She said at that time, the cyst completely drained and never came back. You can also prepare a clay bath by adding four pounds of clay, pouring very slowly , at the point of the faucet, into the running warm water to keep the clay particles from sticking together. Stay in the tub for 20-25 minutes, then stand up, and rinse yourself under the shower. Do not drain the tub just yet. This clay solution must sit for a little time (not more than three or four hours) in order to settle to the bottom. At this point you have several choices. You can now drain the tub, which is not recommended because that would clog the drain. It's better to skim off the surface water and pour it down the sink. When you're finished, compost it or toss it into your yard___after skimming the water, you may want to take a peek at the clay. Some people say that the clay at the bottom of the bathtub changes color. Sometimes becoming a dark brown or black. This is a supposed result of the absorbed and adsorbed toxins. Others say that you should not handle the leftover clay with your hands; instead, you should use rubber gloves when scooping it out . I personally, have a bath-tub outside (we live in a rural area with no immediate neighbors and it is fenced with privacy) I fill the tub with dirt and add water to it to make a nice thick mud paste. Then I'd submerge myself for a few hours or as long as I could. (again, be selective as where you get the dirt).

A friend of ours who lived in Las Vegas, Nevada (Judy) had surgery on her foot and during the course of her healing, the foot didn't heal well. She was in constant pain and taking pain medications, and she was walking with the assistance of a walker. She asked me what I thought she should do, and I naturally explained to her the mud therapy treatment. The next few days, after returning to Las Vegas, I brought some dirt from the desert area and added some good water to form a thick clay, and I put it into a large bucket where she could immerse her entire foot into it. She told me that she followed the instructions and she did this daily for about a week, and would sit outside in the sunshine a few hours a day, with her foot constantly submerged in the cold mud. (cold mud is good for swelling)

She later called me and said she relocated to Kansas. She also told me that she had no more problems with her foot, and was walking normally with no pain.

I, myself have personally used the mud therapy treatments on my own body on many occasions. I make sure the soil is relatively clean with no known impurities(the best of my knowledge) I use clay that is usually located in the desert...not surface city soil, etc. (I usually dig deep into the ground)

At one time I apparently wasn't drinking enough water and my right kidney became inflamed (1998) so I performed the mud treatment on myself. My husband accompanied me out into the desert and I actually did lie down into the dirt and he applied the mud to my kidney area and I remained out there for an hour or so. He remained there with me just in case a snake decided to slither by. We later returned home and I showered, drank water and fresh juiced cranberries (I always buy an excess of fresh cranberries during the thanksgiving season and freeze them. Most bottled cranberry juices have a great deal of added sugar).

I noticed that by the next day the soreness had began to fade, and by the third day, the pain was all gone. During this time, I also didn't eat any red meats. I drank the blended aloe-vera plant (one large leaf) daily, and consumed only healthy fruits and vegetables...avoiding citrus fruits. I also took the recommended doses of liquid Echinacea (?) I **juiced** many fruits and vegetables also.. Parsley, apples and broccoli, and I drank a large amount of water to flush my system...

In May, 2000, I accidentally poked my gums with a sharp object trying to dislodge a piece of food stuck between a tooth. It unfortunately became

Slightly infected. My jaw was beginning to swell and I couldn't eat solid foods on that particular side. I rinsed with peroxide. However, couple of days went by and I thought of the mud (clay treatment) I went outside and gathered a nice clump of clay and added a small amount of water to it and blended an aloe vera leaf, and made it into a paste, then applied a small clump into my mouth onto the affected area. It hurt for a few minutes, but later the pain began to subside. I left it in my mouth for approximately three hours. During this time I was lying outside in the sunshine. In a few hours the pain and swelling began to disappear, and by the next day it was practically gone. By the 3rd day it was gone entirely. During this time, I didn't swallow any of the mud,(because of the extracted toxins) but would

21

expel any excess saliva as it gathered in my mouth. ....At the final end to the procedure, I rinsed thoroughly with water and then actually applied straight aloe vera leaf to the gum area, and left it on for a few minutes.

I believe that God has put healing methods all around us, and we are surrounded by natural medicines and cures untapped by man.

I once started developing a stye on my lower inner eyelid of my right eye. By the end of the day, it had become quite uncomfortable. By the next day it had began to swell and it appeared that I had a black eye.(2008) Actually it started as I was obtaining research for this book.)

I immediately ceased from any further eye-strain (reading, computer work, etc.)

I then applied some **Red- Desert** clay **into** the eye itself with a q-tip and went outside and sat in the sunshine for a few hours. I then rinsed the mud from my eye. In a few hours the swelling began going down and by the next day, the stye had completely disappeared. I also applied warm compresses followed by cold compresses to my eye during the night. (warm to cold) It also helped in reducing the discomfort.

I also read that clay is beneficial for cataracts also.(*be sure to use safe and prepared clay)*

Another testimony was from a woman suffering from cataracts who used pascalite clay in the form of eye drops.(water filtered through pascalite as eye drops.) She reported that the treatment was effective. The cataracts dissolved. Two other people have reported similar results with eye cataracts.

A very close relative, A. Traylor told me that a slice

of raw white potato applied to the eye relieves the discomfort of styes also.

Always remember, when you use clay, it usually takes a few days for the situation to entirely clear up. However, you will feel better even after the first use with the clay at the end of the first day. You also have to do *your part* in the healing process by utilizing healthy habits during the period of illness, etc. Healing is always quicker when the body is being treated well. (herbs, water, rest, etc.

For instance, when I had the stye on my eyelid, I immediately ceased from long periods on the computer, and other types of serious eye-strain situations. I also applied the warm to cold compresses on the eye every chance I could, especially at night.

Scripture reference:

John 9:1-11,
And as Jesus passed by, he saw a man which was blind from his birth.
2 And his disciples asked him, saying, Master, who did sin, this man, or his parents, that he was born blind?
3 Jesus answered, *Neither hath this man sinned, nor his parents; but that the works of God be made manifest in him.*
4 *I must work the works of him that sent me, while it is day: the night cometh, when no man can work.*
5 *As long as I am in the world, I am the light of the world.*
6 When he had this spoken, he spat on the ground, and made *clay* of the spittle, and he anointed the eyes of the blind man with the *clay,*

7 And said unto him, *Go, wash in the pool of Siloam,* (which is interpretation, Sent) He went his way therefore, and washed, and came seeing.

8 The neighbors therefore, and they which before had seen him that he was blind, said, Is not this he that sat and begged?

9 Some said, This is he: others said, He is like him: but he said, I am <u>he.</u>

10 Therefore said they unto him, How were thine eyes opened?

11 He answered and said, A man that is called Jesus made *clay,* and anointed mine eyes, and said unto me, *Go to the pool of Siloam, and wash:* and I went and washed, and I received sight.

<u>(If you notice, **Jesus did choose** to apply *CLAY* to the blind man's eyes...*as a point of contact)*......</u>

Now Na-a--man, captain of the host of the king of Syria, was a great man with his 2 Kings 5:1-14 master, and honorable, because by him the Lord had given deliverance unto Syria: he was also a mighty man in valour, *but he was* a leper.

2 And the Syrians had gone out by companies, and had brought away captive out of the land of Israel a little maid and she waited on Na-a-man's wife.

3 And she said unto her mistress, Would God my Lord *were* with the prophet that *is* in Samaria! For he would recover him of his leprosy.

4 And *one* went in, and told his lord, saying, Thus and thus said the maid that is of the land of Israel.

5 And the king of Syria said, Go to, go, and I will send

a letter unto the king of Israel. And he departed, and took with him ten talents of silver, and six thousand *pieces* of gold, and ten changes of raiment. $52,800 . $384,000 . shekels

6 And he brought the letter to the king of Israel, saying, Now when this letter is come unto thee, behold, I have therewith went Na-a-man my servant to thee, that thou mayest recover him of his leprosy.

7 And it came to pass, when the king of Israel had read the letter, that he rent his clothes, and said, Am I God, to kill and to make alive, that this man doth send unto me to recover a man of his leprosy? Wherefore consider, I pray you, and see how he seeketh a quarrel against me.

8 And it was so, when Elisha the man of God had heard that the king of Israel had rent his clothes, that he sent to the king, saying, Wherefore has thou rent thy clothes? Let him come now to me, and he shall know that there is a prophet in Israel.

9 So Na-a-man came with his horses and with his chariot, and stood at the door of the house of Elisha.

10 And Elisha sent a messenger unto him. Saying,"Go and wash in the Jordan seven times, and thy flesh shall come again to thee, and thou shall be clean".

11 But Na-a-man was wroth, and went away, and said, Behold, I thought, He will surely come out to me, and stand, and call on the name of the Lord his God, and strike his hand over the place, and recover the leper.

12 Are not Abana and Pharpar, rivers of Damascus, better than all the waters of Israel? May I not wash in them, and be clean? So he turned and went away in a rage.

13 And his servants came near, and spake unto him, and said, My father, if the prophet had bid thee do some great thing, wouldst thou not have done it? How much rather then, when he saith to thee, Wash, and be clean?

14 Then went he down, and dipped himself seven times in the Jordan, according to the saying of the man of God: and his flesh came again like unto the flesh of a little child, and he was clean.

Note: The Jordan River is a **MUDDY** river) and Na-a-man was angry because he wanted to dip in a nice clean river of Damascus, and not a muddy one)

(Again, a type of **muddy** solution, etc. was used).

One commentator who visited the Jordan river stated that "It looked like a muddy creek on my dad's farm after a big rain."   (Tammy)

Reflecting @ The Jordan River, By Becky Garrison

Another viewer of the River Jordan stated that it was "akin" to a slow moving muddy stream.

According to the geography of the Jordan River, it is located in Northern Israel and it flows south through the sea of Galilee to the Dead Sea.

In the bible, the Jordan was also the scene of the baptism of Jesus by John the Baptist.

(only our **Lord Jesus Christ** knows why **He** chose to use **mud** ,etc. for **his** point of contact in these healing processes).

God wants us well, and wants us to be healthy and strong in the areas of our lives.

He wants us to be free from the bondages of pain, and sickness. Jesus died for us that we could be well.

He was raised in life, ever making intercessions for us now so that we can be well. And he wants us to strong and healthy, as a witness of His love, His grace, and His power.

"For I will restore health unto thee, and I will heal thee of thy wounds, saith the Lord" (Jeremiah 30:-17)

note: Everyone gets the same amount of time, but no one gets the same results.....

How you treat everyday illnesses that come upon you is your decision. I first confess my healing through Jesus Christ, then I use the natural healing methods and remedies God has placed before me..

Remember, God Wants You Well.

Exodus 15:26 states :

If thou wilt diligently hearken to the voice of the Lord thy God, and wilt do that which is right in his sight, and wilt give ear to his commandments, and keep all his statutes, I will put none of these diseases upon thee, which I have brought upon the Egyptians for *I am the Lord that healeth thee.* "

Remember, the Lord desires for us to eat healthy and to maintain healthy lifestyles also, and it is not His intention to cause diseases to come upon us. It is usually you and I who allow these things to happen by our deliberate unhealthy lifestyles However, if a disease or illness does attack our body, God has provided us with natural remedies and well as **medical doctors.**

note: please contact your physician for all medical matters and pray also to our heavenly Father ---God through His Precious Son, Jesus Christ... for Divine healing in all areas of your body....

27

Preferred clay poultices I found effective:***

Cactus root, pounded to a paste, then added to the moist clay (prickly pears)… with the prickly spines removed then the flesh of the cactus also applied to the affected area. Leave this on until the clay becomes dry and hard. Then discard the used clay. During this procedure, the clay actually draws the toxins from your body. You should do this procedure in the direct sunlight for best results. However, if you don't have sunlight, you do what is best. If it is a rainy day, etc. and has to done indoors, you can used a bathtub lined with plastic, etc… you can improvise to your own preference.

I personally bathe first with a good natural soap that is free of additives, and rinse off completely, then proceed with the mud bath.

If you are bothered with dry skin, make sure that after you bathe with the clay, wait an hour or so(if possible) then apply a light oil on your skin to replace the oils washed away. I commonly use an extra virgin olive oil. (You can use a natural oil of your preference).

By waiting for a brief period of time you let your body absorb the water from the bath (like a sponge), then add the oil to seal the moisture into your skin. If you add oil too early, the slick coating on your skin will seal the moisture out. **Also drink plenty of good water.** An adequate amount replenishes or dehydrates your cells.

If your live in a climate with high humidity, be thankful and enjoy it. Do you ever notice how people in the tropics generally have beautiful skin? You see less dryness. Today, many people suffer from dry skin due to constant exposure to air-conditioned homes, _clay with ground olive leaf_

cars and offices. Heating lowers the amount of relative humidity in the air, and air-conditioning actually removes moisture. Usually you can't control the humidity levels in your workplace, but you can alter the air at home. Room humidifiers are efficient and cost relatively little. Also, ask your air conditioning/heating contractor about adding a whole house humidifier to your central heating and air system.

Favorite poultices(continued)

Clay with ground olive leaves…for external infections
Clay with blended aloe vera leaves ..for external as well as internal usages
I also take adequate amounts of vitamin C and also liquid calcium.*****
Echinacea is also good to take. I enjoy the liquid, however, you can take the capsules available at your local health food store) It helps to jump start your immune system.

Other applications of clay:

*Apply clay mixed with aloe vera to burns, sunburns and scalds. It will relieve the pain. Make a paste and apply. Clay mixed with slippery elm tea….makes a wonderful poultice as a _drawing_ poultice for boils and splinters. Native Americans used the bark of the slippery elm when it was beaten to a pulp, to treat gunshot wounds and help remove bullets.
For insect bites and stings, make a paste (poultice)

Clay and myrrh (herb) prepared with a tea made

from the boiled flowers of sunflowers .
It will relieve the pain and draw out the poison.
Clay and Frankincense (herb) also makes a
wonderful poultice for drawing out toxins.

Circulatory problems:

The heart and the Blood

According to **Michael Abehsara**, the author of the **Healing Clay,** clay is rich in diastases (enzymes) which account for its ability to fix free oxygen and purify and enrich the blood. Free radicals are atoms whose electrons have been stripped; and which a certain number of them are necessary to stave off invading bacteria. An excess can attack the body, causing cellular breakdown. Clay contributes to an improved blood supply.

High levels of blood risk factors, such as too many free radicals, help to explain the breakdown of the cardiovascular system in the form of strokes or heart attacks. If the body system continues to pump dirty blood to the heart, heart disease is sure to follow. The vessel walls are eventually weakened by weak blood, which cannot carry the nutrients needed for blood vessel reinforcement. Clays cleansing action on the stomach, small intestine, and colon may prevent this. The suggested dosage is 1-2 level tablespoons once or twice per day, taken together with fiber (psyllium seed, apple pectin, or guar gum) Fiber, too is known to reduce the level of cholesterol in the blood. Like the clay, it binds to the bile.

Clay has also been found beneficial in treating hemorrhoids, menstrual cramps, prostrate problems in men, arthritis, chronic fatique syndrome, gum disease,(gingivitis and pyorrhea) headache, syphilis and diarrhea.

Female yeast infections: (Clay can be used vaginally or anally)

There have been documented facts that clay has also been beneficial in treating yeast infections. (be sure to use safe clay that has preferably been purchased.)

Also mix it with *adequate (runny(* **water before administering it into those areas.+**

Additional uses:

Add clay to water for its purification properties. According to **Ran Knishinsky,** the author of **The Clay Cure** when he visits Mexico, he takes along with him a jar of clay and adds a pinch or two to every glass of water he drinks. (for the prevention of dysentery)

Add clay powder to your dog's or cat's water bowl.

Also can be given to other farm animals.(horses, cattle, etc.)

Clay minerals provide an excellent source of nutrients for potted plants, and also adsorb many free mineral ions in the soil___add to the soil freely.

Note: *The spiritual leader,* **Mahatma Gandhi** *praised clay for a multitude of uses.*

I recently read a testimonial of a woman who told how the terramin clay actually helped her tremendously with Carpal Tunnel Syndrome. By her testimony, she began taking a teaspoon of terramin clay in the morning with a glass of water, and she said it took approximately one month faithfully for her to feel the actual results from the clay. You can read her testimonal on her website: *Live2ski2@aol.com*

Other clay poultices:

Use prepared clay and add your favorite tea for the binder: St. Johns wort, yellow dock, or horsetail. You can also use rosemary and basil. Apply this mixture to the affected area at least every 3-4 hours. Cover the area and lie on a plastic protective covering. (to protect your bedlinens) Let this mixture remain on overnight (or as long as-- is convenient for you. It can be a longer or shorter time period, however, the longer- the better...

Clay Masque:

The clay facial masque deep cleans pores, exfoliates dead cells, and leaves the skin feeling soft and clean. It stimulates skin circulation and has an astringent action on sagging tissues. The facial muscles become toned from the application of the clay masque. You may wish to use clay alone when preparing a masque, or mix it with several other ingredients of your choice. One of my favorite formulas consists of three ounces of clay, one banana peel (ground) outer rind of a pineapple, mango, kiwano and persimmon. Also use ground almonds, honey and lemon juice. Blend all of these ingredients together and add to the clay mixture. Store these mixtures into a *glass* container in the refrigerator and use as needed.

Psoriasis has been relieved by the treatment of clay also. (Make a paste of clay **and aloe vera, let dry and rinse it off.**)

Poison ivy has also been treated with success by making a poultice of cactus root (pounded to a paste) and clay . Apply to the affected area, let dry and rinse it off.

Clay is also beneficial to **poison ivy** by mixing it with

sassafras root bark, made into a tea. (it is also very good as a warming tea to drink). Sassafras has been used for treating high blood pressure, rheumatism, arthritis, gout, and kidney problems.

We personally drink the tea on a regular basis. It is a wonderful beverage served hot with honey. My children were raised on it, and I would greet them with a cup of sassafras tea with honey when they would get home from school on cold, wintery days. You can actually find the actual sassafras tree growing in many wooded areas in the *southern* United States and the tea is available in most health food stores. When the actual bark or root is boiled, the water turns to a beautiful red color, and you can boil the same piece of root or bark many times before the color dissipates.

Poison Sumac:

The leaves of **Ragweed** are also crushed, mixed with clay and applied to the infected areas of the skin.

The herb ragweed is listed in 1983 British Herbal Pharmacopoeia for **skin diseases**, rheumatic problems and gout.

Clay and liniment plasters of chest discomfort:

Apply a warm poultice or plaster of clay mixed with a tea made from the boiled branches and stems of the Scots *Pine Tree.*

Scots pine has quite a wide range of medicinal usages, being valued especially for its antiseptic action and beneficial effect upon the respiratory system. It may be used in cases of bronchitis, sinusitis or upper respiratory problems. Scots Pine branches and stems yield a thick resin, which is also antiseptic within the respiratory tract.

I make pine tree tea on a regular basis by boiling the pine needles and small branches and adding honey. It is very warming to the system.

My daughter, Deborah had a very severe headache at one time, and I gave her a cup of pine needle tea with honey and mint, and she said it relieved the headache.

Also use the herb *feverfew* for headaches.(made into a tea) It relieved a migraine headache Deborah had also. It also relaxes tension; just boil the herb and drink it plain or with honey. If you have severe migrains, pack cool clay around your temples (head and scalp areas) to assist in relieving the swelling and pressure that occurs during the migraine itself;) remember, clay does draw out extra fluid.(swelling,(edema) as the result of traumatic blows or pain, which is also attributed to swelling around the injured site.

Mud Baths:

These treatments have a very long and interesting usage. Cleopatra used black mud bath therapy to enhance her complexion. Today, a mud bath is the most wanted treatment in many places in the country.

The mixture of mud helps to cleanse the pores in the skin. It revitalizes the skin and makes it soft and shiny. The mud bath also offers numerous health benefits.

The mud- bath treatment is more effective than any other treatment. It provides great relaxation from stress and offers a unique experience. It grants warm feelings of being covered with a shelter of soft mud. The warm temperature helps to cleanse the dirt in the skin leaving it soft and supple. The natural ingredients in mud bath helps to get rid of muscular pain and joint pains.

Mud bathing also helps to remove blackheads and blemishes in the facial skin. It acts as an anti aging property and helps to maintain the elasticity of the skin. It has skin detoxification properties and so it removes all harmful toxins from the skin. Since it absorbs more water, it retains the hydration in the skin and makes it soft. It induces the skin to absorb the essential nutrients in the mud.

The quality mud -bath is used for both health and cosmetic purposes. It shows significant improvement in curing rheumatoid arthritis. It also helps to treat various skin diseases. Hence, it is the most required treatment nowadays.

Mud specially prepared by utilizing rich bio- minerals has anti-inflammatory properties and so it is able to decrease inflammation. The users therefore experience great relief from irritation, swelling or minor skin problems. It also helps to reduce muscular pains and stress. It has the capacity to treat dry skin conditions. The balanced mixture of bio minerals in the mud helps to improve blood circulation and thereby treats various health problems.

Mud -bathing is the simplest method of rejuvenating the entire body. I personally use it on a monthly basis, (or whenever it is convenient) especially when it is warm outside. (We live outside of the city limits where we have a fenced in yard with privacy; therefore I have my own private tub, (nothing elaborate, just an old bath-tub) where I can take mud baths at my leisure.) I also incorporate many other herbs into the bath also like mint, papaya, capsum, cornsilk, Echinacea, seaweed as well as others.

If you don't have access to a backyard tub, and you desire (or need) to take a mud bath, you can do it in your own bathtub **or** you can call your local state directory and locate a beauty - spa , (etc) that does mud baths...

If you decide to take a mud bath in your own bathtub, in the clean-up process, you might consider using a dustpan to scrape it up from tub afterwards. (Again you weigh the inconvenience to the necessity of the issue; and that is your health.) I also apply mud on my hair and scalp...(although this can be messy) just rinse you hair **thoroughly!** I usually do this procedure outside.

After shampooing and rinsing your hair, *mix clay* and a tea made from boiled rosemary leaves and branches, and apply this mixture to your hair, and scalp. Leave it on for at least one hour, then rinse thoroughly with warm rosemary infused water. Rosemary is considered one of the strongest natural antioxidants. It also increases circulation, reduces headaches and fight bacterial and fungal infections. Rosemary contains many compounds that are reported to prevent the breakdown of acetylcholine in the brain, usually a symptom of Alzheimer's disease. Several, if not all can be absorbed through the skin.

As a warming herb, it stimulates circulation of blood to the head, improving concentration and memory. It eases headaches and migraine, and encourages **hair growth by improving blood flow to the scalp.** (A friend of mine I met from Israel stated that they used Rosemary tea for female problems also)

Herbs Usages S-T, Nutritional Research Center
(Again, you will do what you feel is necessary...no matter what the cost!!!!

There are also many other types of clay detox bathing

procedures. (see the end of this book for phone numbers, etc.) Certain clay baths have been specifically prepared for the removal of environmental pollutants, dental/mercury, detox, smokers/ drug detox, arsenic, aluminum, copper and lead, formaldehyde, and *radiation* (Health care providers working in oncology units of hospitals should take these detox baths, also if you've been exposed to *radiation.*, such as x-rays, etc. (however, this silent killer is everywhere present and we are daily exposed to it and in our atmosphere.)

External uses:

After washing your face with the clay mixture, rinse your face with warm water then splash on cold water to close pores. Wait until your face is dry, then apply a thin film of natural moisturizing oil or cream . (use one of your choice)

Psoriasis: Nell C. of Amboy Washington stated that Pascalite clay cured her **psoriasis**. She had used other things prior but with no results. However, she purchased a pound of Pascalite clay, mixed it with water to make a thich paste and applied it to the areas. When it dried, she washed it off with warm water and applied peroxide with a cotton ball.. After it dried she repeated the same treatment during the night -hours and wrapped her legs in plastic and let it dry more gradually. She began this treatment in May of 1970 and continued through to August. and she didn't have a scar left.

If you only have a shower, you can use **Pascalite** in foot and shin detoxes by using a wide shin- high pail that both legs can fit into. I have also used this remedy by putting the pail on the floor in front of me while I spend time on the computer.(keeping my feet submerged, and afterwards having another pail of clear water and a towel to rinse and dry my feet)

Mud baths have been a tradition in Calistoga since the time of Maya Camas Indians. It was formed after a series of volcanic eruptions 2-6 million years ago. They are geothermal waters rich in magnesium and calcium that burst gently into steaming pools and rivers. Calistoga is found at the foot of Mt. St. Helens in the Napa Valley. **The combination of mineral water from the local springs are from Mt. St. Helena make up the key components of the Calistoga Mud.**

Teeth and Gums:

I have also used clay and sage leaves for a toothpaste and gum treatment. After brushing gently with a small amount of clay (all gravel removed) rinse, and rub fresh sage and peppermint leaves over your teeth and gums,with your index finger. As you do this you can actually feel and hear the "squeaky" clean sounds of your teeth and gums; Then rinse thoroughly with cool water. It will leave your mouth feeling wonderful, fresh and clean.(I have personally done this.)

Pascalite Clay has also been found to be effective with **pyorrhea** by applying cotton pads soaked with the clay and applied between the gums and cheeks.

One woman stated that her dentist advised her to get all of her teeth removed due to severe gum disease(pyorrhea) so she began applying the cotton pads soaked with pascalite to her teeth and gums and the infection eventually disappeared.

Also make sure you are taking enough calcium/

Clay & saye ⊳ Toothpaste

magnesium during this time as well as taking a **good strong laxative** and having very good bowel elimination habits to keep your body system free of the gum or tooth infection)

Penile Herpes Simplex:

One person testified that when he applied pascalite clay mixed with honey and applied it to the affected area, within three days the swelling had disappeared and within a few weeks, it had disappeared altogether; when it re-appeared the following year, he applied pascalite and water and it again disappeared.

There was another testimony told to me personally by a friend(Cecilia L) that she used the herb Wild Yam (cream) for a severe burn discoloration. She said she used it faithfully for a few months and the scar disappeared.

She also stated that she rubbed the cream (wild yam)between both thighs, the middle of her back and near the rib-cage, which prevented her from having hot-flashes during the menopausal period. She said she never had them. (wild yam can be purchased at your local health food stores.)

Deodorant:

You can use it by applying dry clay to underarms as well as the bottom of your feet.(Radishes can be crushed and used also mixed with the clay for smelly feet) the plant contains raphanin, which is antibacterial.

I have personally used the dry clay as a deodorant, and it works. I have been unable for years to use regular deodorant because it causes me to get sore areas under my arms. A close relative, Jobie F. said she used rubbing alcohol to clean the armpits well and refrained from using deodorant. I found that helped also. However, under certain circumstances, I now apply the dry clay also and it really works well.

Foot soaks: in mud are wonderful for tired feet as well as some foot disorders. Use cold mud and mix with tumeric spice, which is an anti-inflammatory agent. (*tumeric spice will often stain your clothing or skin area slightly orange when using it in a poultice). (tumeric is also used for foot inflammation)*

Use clay and fresh ground mint leaves for tired feet. (use cool clay) as preferred.

It is especially good on sprains, and helps your body mend more quickly as well as giving physical relief from pain and discomfort. You can use a large bucket or container to submerge your entire foot. The colder the mud, the better it is for the swelling. (edema) (It is convenient to have another bucket of clean, warm water close by to rinse your feel off, as well as a few clean, large towels to dry them off).

I complete the mud treatment with a cool mineral water foot bath and a soothing foot massage (if medically possible) with the actual leaves of a peppermint or spearmint plant.(again if there are no fractures, etc.) **
*At this point, **always** check with your physician if you are unsure of a **possible** fracture or something more serious.*

I've found that a few general procedures administered can be beneficial in avoiding some potential health problems. They are:

1. Eat healthy (as possible)
2. Don't consume **too much** of one thing on a

consistent basis(except water)

3. Be moderate in all eating habits

4. Try to avoid large amounts of prepared food. Such as lunch-meats, T. V. Dinners, etc.

5. Drink plenty of water (6-8 glasses per day)

6. Get plenty of rest.

7. Maintain good elimination habits (very important)

Hippocrates stated: "Your food shall be your medicine and your medicine shall be your food."

Whatever we consume into our body is used for growth, upkeep (maintenance) and repair. That is how food acts as a medicine. The body must also assimilate the foods consumed to receive their vital nutritional elements. When food enters the small intestine, the pancreas and small bowel wall must send juices and bile to individually digest the carbohydrates, proteins and fat. That's a lot of work for a healthy system; much more so for one that is already sick. If the body cannot perform this job then the cells become weakened and starve. Eventually, they will die.

Resting your body and mind is also of great importance. A friend I met a few years ago (Elaine V.) was an older woman and had been married to a medical doctor who had been one of the first founders of a major hospital in the Los Angeles area. She told me that her parents had a large retail business while she was growing up as a young girl, and they always took a 15 minute break every few hours while they were working, just to rest. She said they both lived to be into their late nineties. A glass of <u>red wine cider </u>is also beneficial at night before going to bed. It also has many relaxing qualities for the body. (in moderation always)

I found that in **normal** situations, if you keep your mind and body busy with constructive work and activity during the day, you will be ready for sleep and it **normally** comes naturally. However, there are times when you might have something on your mind that is pressing and it is more difficult to fall asleep. I *first pray and meditate on the goodness of God and ask Him to help me **sleep.*** . Then I will sometimes have a cup of hot herbal tea to relax my mind and body. you can also add an ounce or two of natural red wine cider to your tea. (if desired)

A great recipe I have for homemade cider(is as follows:)

I obtained this recipe from Mrs. Europe J. of Mississippi one very hot summer afternoon. (1990)

She was a small, lovely Afro-American lady who was very alert and was 86 years of age at the time, and lived alone in a small country home, which she kept in immaculate condition. It was very hot -that particular summer day; approximately 105 degrees f; and she served us a glass of homemade wine cider that was simply delicious. It was as clear as apple cider. She later gave me the recipe, and said it was given to her by her grandmother.

The recipe was as followed:

2-½ gallons *good* water (that is what she called it)
2-½ pounds of natural sugar
One package dry yeast
fruit
(ripe fruit of your choice that contain adequate pectin (peaches, plums apples grapes etc.) leave the peelings

on as well as the seeds not removed All of these add to the flavor. (even stems if desired) (I personally leave them on__especially grapes. (I don't measure the fruit, however, just enough to have your container at least ¾ full of the fruit .) I also mash the fruit or grapes (you can use the blender also by just pulsing to assist in breaking down the fruit, especially grapes and smaller fruits where it is difficult to free the juices...) (remember in Italy, they crush the grapes with their feet; however you do whatever procedure that is best for you... (I use the blender). you can use any fruit you desire (just experiment) Always use a large glass or crock container(at least 4-5 gallon container..**I bought a few from a local store**)   **IT CANNOT BE PLASTIC! A PLASTIC** CONTAINER **WILL RUIN YOUR WINE/CIDER.**

Put all of these ingredients into your crock or container, and store it into a dark area(closet, or dark area, etc.) covered loosely with a top, etc. or whatever you have available and let it sit (undisturbed) for seven days. At the end of the seven days, strain it into a colander and cheesecloth... and at that point, add more sugar to your taste and then bottle... **again...only in glass bottles. It's best to use a screw -on cap and don't fill the bottle too full. If you use a cork, be prepared to hear <u>gunshot sounds</u> during the second night It will be the built-up pressure of the wine and the corks will pop off....you will also have wine all over your walls. I've learned that lesson by personal experience.**

According to the article, **The Healing Power of Wine , by Peter Jaret**

"Drink a glass of wine after your soup," an old Russian proverb says, "and you steal a ruble from the doctor." It's a sentiment that nutrition researchers now toast with a raised glass.

You've probably heard that drinking a glass or two of wine a day can lower your risk of dying from heart disease by 30 to 40 percent, according to Harvard University scientist **Walter Wilett**, author of **Eat, Drink and be Healthy** and one of the country's leading nutrition experts. But wine benefits go further: Howard university Hospital researchers reported that moderate wine drinkers are less likely to develop macular degeneration, an age-related eye condition that can lead to partial blindness. Other recent studies suggest postmenopausal women who **consume moderate** amounts of alcohol every day__ __the equivalent of one to two glasses of wine___have stronger bones than non-drinkers. Wine may also lower risk of diabetes and gallstones.

How does wine bestow its remarkable benefits? In the case of heart disease, researchers shows that alcohol opens up arteries and increases blood flow. That's important, since a heart attack usually occurs when a blood clot robs heart muscles of oxygen. **Moderate** drinking also increases levels of HDL cholesterol____so called good cholesterol___which helps the body get rid of LDL cholesterol, the artery clogging form. The antioxidants abundant in some forms of alcohol, especially red wine, can prevent LDL cholesterol from oxidizing.; this damages artery walls, setting the stage for heart disease. But remember, says **Willett,** "there are plenty of ways to get many of the same benefits." Exercise and a better diet top the list. If you do drink, remember a piece of old age wisdom: **moderation in all things.** Beyond two or three drinks a day, the risks begin outweighing the benefits;

Maintaining good elimination habits is a must for a healthy body. Your body is like a plumbing system, and you **must** eliminate the toxins that are consumed naturally in your body daily: that is the functions of your colon and kidneys. Kidneys eliminate toxins, therefore, you must drink plenty of water. (if necessary, keep a gallon of water by your bedside.)

If your body fails to rid itself of toxins through the bowels, a constipated condition arises in which the toxins never leave the body. They actually rot and putrefy right there inside of your body. What's worse, the body doesn't know the difference between live food and dead food in the colon. It will try to get nourishment out of waste. This procedure naturally puts a strain to every functioning cell in your body, and you will feel uncomfortable and ill. At times it is felt to be a queasy upset stomach symptom. You can actually feel the difference when your body has healthy elimination habits and when it doesn't.

A friend of ours, Don A.(an evangelist) had developed an infected toe, and to complicate the situation, he was diabetic. His wife, dotty, was quite concerned because the doctor had stated that it was a possibility that the toe might have to be amputated because at this point, it was beginning to turn black, and was extremely painful. Dottie called me and asked me what I thought could be done naturally. (they were aware that I believed in GOD's natural Healing processes.)

At this point I asked Don if he would be willing to do anything necessary for his foot to be healed. He agreed. We began a seven day body detoxe routine of drinking senna tea and eating aloe vera plant leaves…(Dotty told me that he was eating the very bitter aloe stems like they were green -beans) There procedure took seven days, which is Gods number of completion.

His daily routine was as followed:

Recite healing scripture daily
1 Peter 2:24.....Who his own self bare our sins in his own body on the tree, that we, being dead to sins, should live unto righteousness: by whose stripes *ye were healed*.

No red meats (only chicken or fish)
Drink fresh vegetable juices (juiced in a juicer)at least a quart per day. Or more.)
Do not wear a shoe if possible!.....
Soak the foot in mud for 2-3 hours daily...then rinse it off with distilled water.
Elevate the foot on a pillow, expose to the fresh air and sunshine for at least an hour or as long as you can...
Continue to eat the aloe vera plants (leaves) daily (many as you can tolerate) they are very bitter. (you can blend them with fruit juices also)Aloe vera juice can be purchased from the health food store, but I do prefer the fresh one you make for yourself from the actual plant.

He did this procedure faithfully (in a prayerful spirit) and at the end of seven days, his wife called me and said that his toe was back to the normal color and the soreness was gone.

A former nursing supervisor, Bonnie N. (R. N.) told me that when she was a child growing up in Indiana, if she or a family member would experience an injury, or insect sting, her father would tell them to "put some mud on it". This, she said was a common practice there.

I used to get my nails done at a certain shop In Lancaster, Ca. My manicurist was from viet-nam.(pam) She stated that in her country, there were many mushrooms growing wild in the woods. Some Poisonous and some not...however, they all looked the same. Unfortunately, many people had been accidentally poisoned by eating the poisonous variety.

She said that is was an old -fashioned practice that when someone was poisoned,

They were "buried" in a mud pit up to their necks overnight. By the next morning, they were o.k. and the mud had actually drawn out the poison.

Where do Toxins come from?
Toxins come from many sources, a few which include:

1. Drugs
2. Ingredients in cookware, sodas, toothpaste, deodorant, etc.
3. Environmental pollutants in the air we breathe (smoke, fumes, plastics, Industrial chemicals, etc.
4. Food---herbicides, pesticides, food additives and preservatives, msg and many more
5. Mercury amalgam fillings, fish
6. Pesticides and fertilizers we use at home
7. Fermentation from undigested foods consumed
8. Even unhealthy thoughts and emotions

How do I rid my body of these toxins?

Detoxification

to use the method of detoxification; which is where the human body cleanses itself from the inside our of accumulated wastes we encounter each day and releasing them through the elimination channels of the human body. The liver, spleen, kidneys, bowel, lung, skin and lymphatic system performs this function on a daily basis, that is if the diet intake is good and the body is healthy. *(check with your local health food store, and they should have a number of detoxing preparations and formulas for the human body.)*

***it is important to eliminate all wastes from the body every day. If the diet has been less than what is considered "healthy", most likely the organs cells and body systems are functioning less efficiently as they did when we were children.**

Over the years as toxins accumulate, they block the body's ability to absorb nutrients from the food we eat. The body's natural process of detoxification becomes sluggish and the waste cannot be eliminated properly, often leading to the various health challenges we experience daily.

The juice of organic vegetables is rich in nutrients. As the cells of your body are bathed in these fresh, alkaline vegetable juices, they begin to release acids, which are toxins that can be removed through the elimination channels of the body. Juicing provides a rich source of live enzymes essential to the digestive process. Enzymes are proteins that break down foods into nutrients your body can readily digest. When you eat, digestive enzymes are released from your saliva glands sending signals to the stomach and small intestine in preparation for digestion.

Adults have usually used up all of their digestive enzymes by the time they are 30 and often earlier due to the **SADD** diet which is the **"Standard American Daily Diet". (fast foods, etc.)** Often, people will take digestive enzymes when they eat for this very reason.... to aid in digesting.

It is vital to detoxify the body when treating deficiencies. If the body is toxic and nutrients are taken in whether from foods or supplements, the nutrients will not be able to be absorbed very well. For example, if a sponge is full of dirty water (as the cells are full of toxins), adding additional water to the sponge will have little impact, even if the water is clean.

"THE TRUTH IS THAT NUTRITIONAL DEFICIENCIES AND TOXICITY GO HAND IN HAND. IF YOU TREAT DEFICIENCIES WITHOUT ADDRESSING TOXICITY YOU MAKE LITTLE HEADWAY AND LIKEWISE, IF YOU TREAT TOXICITY WITHOUT ADDRESSING DEFICIENCIES THEN NO LONG-TERM BENEFIT WILL APPLY".

***Therefore, juicing will assist in breaking down toxins, cleanse the body, carry oxygen and nutrients directly to the cells and tissues, and allow nutrients to be better absorbed.

Certain juices can Detoxify your body. They are:
Green vegetables:

Spinach
Parsley
Celery
Swiss chard
Kale
Endive
Cabbage(drink immediately)
Beets and tops
Carrots and tops if they are freshly grown (We grow
most of our own)

Use vegetables of your choice...make sure it is organic
(if possible) and wash thoroughly with a vegetable brush.
(It is not difficult to grow your own vegetables in your
yard, or on a balcony in a pot: just replace a few flowers
for vegetables.)

Cilantro and Mung beans are excellent heavy metal
removers as well. (you can grow these from your home
quite easily)

After the juice is made, it can be transferred to the
blender to add Spirulina and flax seed oil. Be sure to buy
an organic brand of spirulina , which is a high source of
anti-oxidants. Check with your health provider to get a
good brand . Remember to put **Himalayan Crystal Salt**
on your tongue for the benefit of stimulating the body to
absorb more nutrients. you can also use **Celtic** salt .

**(Maryanne Maldonado) A wellness coach in the
Arizona area.....**

A good regime for detoxifying your body is to drink
this vegetable drink twice a day. You can find these salts
at your local health food store.

Can you eat clay?

Of course you can!

I'm sure you've heard that many pregnant women often crave clay, which is probably a certain mineral they are lacking. Remember that the earth itself receives its vital energies from the sun, air, and waters, and is a most powerful healing agent of physical regeneration.

Clay, mud and sand; are all different forms of earth; all participate in life-giving, health restoring processes.

You can even purchase clays that are considered to be pure and of the highest quality. (check your local health food stores, etc.

In the back of this book, I will give you a list of places where to purchase these different clays.

There is a premium calcium montmorillonite clay (Terramin) or red desert clay, or Bentonite.

Bentonite Clay is an effective detoxifier with substances that absorb toxins from our GI tract. Bentonite clay can never be absorbed by the body, so it's not poisonous at all.

According to the law of physics, opposites attract. Therefore, it makes Bentonite Clay very effective in binding to toxins.

The Bentonite clay is like a magnet that attracts toxins. It can absorb any toxic substances imaginable: impurities, harmful bacteria, poisons, pesticides, pathogens, parasites, etc. It does this without posing any side effects in us, because it can't be absorbed by us.

Bentonite Clay ultimately cleans the intestinal linings. After a colon cleanse, the colon can then absorb nutrients and minerals much easier than before. As a result, our symptoms and sicknesses disappear from this boost in absorption, and the elimination of toxins.

Always take any edible clay with some form of fiber. One to use is Psyllium Husk. The fiber will help push the clay out through the intestines, as well as all the toxins it attracts.

Without the basic minerals (calcium, iron, magnesium, potassium, manganese, and silica as well as trace elements, those appearing in very tiny amounts, major deficiencies deficiencies will develop. The lack of either will make it impossible for the body to maintain good health.

Most people fail to realize the importance of minerals and underestimated their use. In most clays, the mineral exists in natural proportion to one another. This encourages their absorption by the intestinal tract. Accordingly, clay has been used by many tribes and cultures in the treatment of anemia and other mineral deficiencies.

Clay works best when it is taken over a long period of time. That's because its actions are subtle. It starts off slowly and then continues to work faster.

As I have stated, clay does not offer "quick fixes" for all ailments but history shows it can encourage the body to put up a better fight when taken over a long period of time.

When clay is taken for indefinite periods of time, it has no addictive qualities. This is a big concern for many who begin eating the clay. The effects can be so positive that it scares them into thinking they might need it the rest of their life.

However, you can stop taking the clay at any time,

and there are no withdrawal symptoms.

It is my opinion that I do intend to attempt to keep my body as healthy as possible for the rest of my life; therefore, why not take whatever it takes to do so. (especially a natural element such as clay that will help clean out the body; especially in today's polluted world) The liver and kidneys are so overworked they never have a chance to rest. Taking a spoonful of earth minerals every day helps them work better and keeps the mind and body functioning in good condition.

(This edible clay will help the body stay in an alkaline state where diseases cannot thrive.)

(**Terramin**) clay also provides an assortment of essential minerals in a highly absorbable form. It is safe, effective, gentle and it stimulates the body systems to heal itself and recover from many ailments.

The habit of eating dirt (clay) has been long assumed to be an attempt to rectify mineral deficiencies in the human diet. It has become apparent that the clay content is often the most important ingredient of selected soils. Clay is an effective binding agent as its chemical structure allows other chemicals to bond with it and so lose their reactivity. Clay is therefore an effective deactivator of toxins from diet or pathogens.

CBS News aired an article on eating clay which might be beneficial for pregnant women

By Marc Lallanilla

October 3, 2005

While most people would recoil at the thought of eating mud or clay, some medical experts say it may be beneficial, especially for pregnant women.

The habit of eating clay, mud or dirt is known as geophagy.

Cultures worldwide have practiced geophagy for centuries, from the ancient Greeks to Native Americans.

Some Native American women often given their infants small pieces of clay to eat in order to pacify them while they were busy doing other things. (Native tradition taught them which clays were edible, while science utilizes modern techniques today to distinguish clay mineral types from the common grain of clay.)

It has been documented that humans have been eating earth for at least forty thousand years. *"Cindy Engles, Ph.D. "*(on every continent except Antartica.

"Every time I get pregnant, I get a craving.....I have to eat it," *Ruth Anne T. Joiner,* 40 who has given birth to four healthy babies.....

It melts in your mouth like chocolate, says Joiner, describing her favorite treat. "The good stuff is real smooth," she adds. "It's like a piece of candy." Joiner is describing the delectable taste of dirt, specifically, clay from the region around her home in Montezuma, Ga.

Though the practice is rarely if ever recommended by medical professionals, some nutritionists now admit the habit of eating clay may have some real health benefits.

"It is possible that the binding effect of clay would cause it to absorb toins, "said Dr. David L. Katz, nutrition expert at the Yale School of Medicine and a medical contributor for ABC News.

Clay's ability to absorb plant toxins is well

documented. Jared Diamond, professor of geography and physiology at the David Geffen School of Medicine at UCLA and author of "Guns, Germs, and Steel: The Fates of Human Societies" has written on clays that are especially good at binding with plant toxins.

Clays and Poisons:

It has been found that clay taken internally can counteract the effects of digested poisons. They noted that the ingested poison, paraquat given to rats, caused respiratory failure, liver damage, and kidney failure, which soon led to death. Several adsorbents were shown to be effective in counteracting the effects of the poison .Among them were bentonite, commonly called montmorillonite. In this experimental situation, clay was given in repeated doses rather than single doses. The effectiveness of repeated doses is apparently due to its ability to prevent the gastrointestinal absorption of paraquat, which can continue up to 30 hours even after injestion in rats. Surprisingly, even when the treatment was delayed for 10 hours after the oral administration of paraquat, the therapy was successful. The rats did not die and toxic damage was minimal.

The authors of the report went on to say that since urinary paraquat levels have been detected for as long as 31 days after ingestion, continued efforts, as well as early efforts, to eliminate absorbed paraquat may be important. Therefore, continual use of the clay is advisable because of its ongoing adsorptive properties. The doctors concluded the article by saying that in case any lethal doses of paraquat are ingested, the clay should be administered as soon as possible. In cases of gastrointestinal poisoning, one teaspoon of clay can be repeated at regular intervals.(every 1-2 hours) up to 48 hours after ingestion. If the case is severe and seious, please call 911 and seek urgent medical assistance...

Note: **Robert Robertson,** author of **Fuller's Earth,** has a very interesting comment on the role of clay as an antidote to poison. He writes:

Although the use of **calcium montmorillonite** as an antidote to poisons has been known for centuries, and the scientific reasons for its success have been known for decades, it is strange that, in a world where heavy metal solutions, alkaloids, cationic pesticides and detergents could be accidentally ingested, this clay is not yet included in first aid boxes and chemical laboratories.

What is cancer: Causes and symptoms:

Note:

Cancerous tissues are acidic at a Ph level of 7.4. Cancer cells become dormant when the Ph level reaches 8.5, cancer cells die

The body is made up of trillions of cells, which divide and multiply as the body needs them. Cancer is the uncontrolled growth of abnormal cells which reproduce usually due to serious weakness of the immune system.

When the immune system is overwhelmed with toxins and not given proper nutrients to maintain health, it ceases to function as nature intended and breaks down allowing for uncontrolled growth of abnormal cells, which can multiply and become cancer.

According to **Jethro Kloss**, the author of **Back to Eden** *cancer has been related to chronic auto-intoxication, constipation, inactivity of all the organs... (the lungs, liver, kidneys, skin and bowels. When there is improper elimination* *of these areas, they become overloaded with toxins, then the poisons accumulate around the weakest organs or where it becomes injured by a blow, fall, or bruise. The poisoning of the body has been caused by the use of tea, coffee, cola drinks, fatty meats and excessive liquor as well as (tobacco) in all forms.*

Fats have been found to promote breast cancer in mice. Hormones are found in breast cancer and the current suspicion is that fats may over-stimulate harmone production or disrupt normal harmone balance.

It has been found that cancer has been on an alarming increase **(1 of 3 persons get cancer).** *Here are a list of things not to do as a method of prevention as well as things to do to keep your body healthy....and also what to do if you do get this disease.*

I'm using this reference to cancer because it is on the rise, and it is mainly due to our unhealthy lifestyles.

I noticed about ten years ago (1990') how children were eating more fast foods on a regular basis; for instance, they were eating fast foods for breakfast, lunch and dinner.

Now, it has become common for children to develop diabetes, as well as many types of cancers also. These same statistics are true with teenagers and adults. Therefore, we are getting to, and have reached *a very sick society*, and unfortunately, society (the media) seems to look the other way when it comes to what we put into our bodies. Everything has to be done quickly now so microwaves does it real fast, but microwaving is also very dangerous to your health.

Instead of preparing good healthy foods, your local fast food establishment is now serving your favorite hot sandwich (usually quite unhealthy) with a soda (also equally unhealthy)

Many people reply to the fast food situation(or fast lifestyles)

"Well, I'm going to die of something, so what!"

However, they don't realize that when they contact a certain disease due to neglect of the body, it *can be - and is usually* accompanied by a great deal of pain or discomfort to themselves, as well as the financial strain brought on to themselves as well as to their families.

Improper foods that contribute to cancer:

Fatty meats (prepared meats, cold cuts, etc.)
White sugar
White flour
<u>**Soft drinks**</u>
 <u>**tobacco uses: (Smoking, etc.)**</u>
(a cancer study implicates coffee agent)
    <u>***The headline of an article from United Press International, Washington, June 18, 1982***</u> showed that a two year study states the result showed a chemical commonly used in decaffeinated coffee causes liver cancer in laboratory mice.

Other Contributing factors:

According to an article in Prevention Magazine, March 1988 Issue states:
The survival of cancer has as much to do with the mental attitude as the extent of the disease.
1. Unforgiveness
2. Unresolved anger
3. Bitterness

Prevention and treatment:

1. Detox your body (see above)
2. Keep a positive, healthy mental attitude
3. Smile and be happy
4..When faced with stressful situations which is *inevitable*, take a moment to relax and deep breathe.

(*A merry heart doeth good like a medicine:* But a broken spirit drieth the bones.

Proverbs 17:22

(I read once about a woman who had been diagnosed with terminal breast cancer who had actually healed herself by drinking at least one gallon of water a day, eliminating all meats, eating only fresh vegetables and ***laughing*** (purposely) at least seven times a day. Remember, laughter (being merry) is healing.

4. Take a **mud bath** at least once a week (more if possible)
5. Maintain a healthy lifestyle...detoxification, etc.
6. Eat plenty of raw fruits and vegetables.
7. No red meats
8. Begin eating clay 2-4 tablespoons per day
9. Do a colon cleanse (keep regular elimination habits)
10. Drink at least 8-10 glasses of water daily.(more if possible)
11. Take a **sea salt bath** at least once a week. (I get my salt from the Dead Sea in Israel) (see references at the back of this book)
12 . Learn how you can effectively keep your digestive tract (especially your colon) clean.
13. Set aside a minimum of 25 minutes in your day for listening to your body through spiritual meditation with

our Heavenly Father and visualization.

14. Work up to 30 minutes or more of light-moderate exercise (walking, swimming, etc., per day.

(if you use these methods on a regular basis, you *can* prevent many illnesses that can happen, and if it already has happened to you, these are ways in which you can *help* your body get back on track.)

Another book to research concerning cancer is (You Can Heal Yourself, By: Louise Hay

Also, Your Body Believes Every Word You Say......By Barbara Levine

Edible Clay for Healing............a program on Red Desert Clay aired on the Discovery channel____the Animal planet_____Date ?

***This clay does the following"

***Boosts the immune system

***Deposits over 60 essential minerals into the body

***The pH is 8.3 (very alkalinizing)

***Acid reflux systems are elleviated

***Abundant in calcium and silica for reversing osteoporosis

***Leaves behind over 60 essential minerals and trace elements

Ran Knishinsky was diagnosed with a ganglion cyst on his wrist. His doctor gave two options___surgery to remove it or **eat clay minerals"** He chose to eat the clay containing earth minerals, with the intention of clearing the problem at the source as opposed to the surgery to remove it for the time being. After eating clay, Ran watched the tumor completely shrink over a two month period until it was completely gone. This is most likely due to the strong ionic charge of the clay, which binds to toxins or poisons which build up and crystallize in a particular area of the body (in this case, the wrist)

Ran Knishinsky also writes that clay is part of his diet and he never skips a day without eating clay. He writes, "When clay is consumed, its vital force is released into the physical body and mingles with the vital energy of the body, creating a stronger, more powerful energy in the host. The natural magnetic action transmit's a remarkable power to the organism and helps to rebuild vital potential through the liberation of latent energy. When the immune system does not function at its best, the clay stimulates the body's inner resources to awaken the stagnant energy. It supplies the body with the available magnetism to run well. Clay is said to propel the immune system to find a new healthy balance and strengthens the body to a point of higher resistance."

Naturally absorbent and extremely gentle on the system, clay can treat ailments affecting digestion, circulation, menstruation, and the liver, skin, and prostate. Clay also remedies symptoms of arthritis, chronic fatigue syndrome, gum diseases, and migraines.

Clay has also been found beneficial in the treatment and cure of other cysts,

i.e. Ganglion and sebaceous cysts.

Remember, there are many different types of clays, from internal to external. Be sure to inquire as to which is used for that specific purpose. There are also different names of clays. Each one is a little different than the other. (in the back of this book, I will list some distributors where you can actually purchase these clays.

What is Bentonite Clay?

Bentonite is a name given to a particular clay that was originally found in Fort Benton, Wyoming, the name given by W.C Knight in 1898. Previously, it was called Taylorite, which was named after William Taylor, who first drew attention to the clay deposits.

It is a clay generated frequently from the alteration of volcanic ash, consisting predominantly of smectite minerals. Smectites are clay minerals. It is used in various forms. (is utilized in the removal of impurities in oils where its adsorptive properties are crucial in the processing of edible oils and fats (soya/palm/.canola oils.) In drinks such as beer, wine and mineral water, and in products like sugar, bentonite is used as a clarification agent.

Clays have been used world wide for thousands of years. Ancient Egyptians used clays for mummification purposes for its purifying powers..

(Industrial Minerals Association, North America)

Calcium Montmorillonite Clay was first discovered in Montmorillon, France in the 1800's, therefore getting the name, Montmorillonite. They also found that many ships sailing from France were known to store clay on board for the treatment of dysentery as well as other medical problems.

Dr. Simon Cohen, N.D

However, there are only a limited number of Calcium Montmorillonite Clay" deposits around the world..

The name **mortmorillonite** is used currectly both as a **group name for all clay minerals with an expanding lattice except vermiculite, and also** as a specific mineral name.

(R. E. Grim: Mineralogy 2nd edition, McGraw-Hill Book Company, New York (1968) 41

Bentonite Chemical Equation: A12O34SiO2H20

Montmorillonite chemical equation: Nao.2Cao.1 A2Si4O10(OH)2(H20)10

Bentonite, a medicinal powdered clay which is also known as montmorillonite, derives from deposits of weathered volcanic ash.

Calcium Montmorillonite Clay has also been used extensively in the treatment of pain, open wounds, colitis, and a variety of other health problems. It has also been used by Native Americans for centuries as an internal and external healing agent. They would use the clay on open wounds and for stomach or intestinal distress. The key to these benefits is the natural form in which these minerals are found.

Calcium Montmorillonite Clay is in the smectite group of clays. Only the clays within the smectite group have the ability to adsorb. Its unique ability to grow and change (adsorb) is the reason for its classification and recognition as a "Living Clay". While there is more than one Mortmorillonite, the red "**Calcium Montmorillonite Clay**"of the smectite group is a favorite for human use internally and externally.

Clay which has been hydro-thermally altered and seasoned in the arid desert is rich in content. The color of clay is determined by the mixture and ratio of elements within it. Hydrothermal exposures over long periods of time affect the clay in two important aspects; it becomes negatively charged and crystallized. As a result of the crystallization process the clay is reduced into small particles that make it easy for the body to assimilate. The negative charges on the clay give it the ability to adsorb or attract positively charged toxic matter, which is then adsorbed into the clay and dispelled from the body as waste.

(I often put a few tablespoons of clay into my dogs food during times of diarrhea, etc.)

Calcium Montmorillonite Clay is reported to contain at least 67 minerals. They include calcium, iron, magnesium, potassium, manganese, and silica as well as trace elements, those appearing in very tiny amounts. Without the basic minerals, major deficiencies will develop. The lack of either will make it impossible for the body to maintain good health.

Most people are not aware of the importance of minerals and underestimated their use. By people being deficient in these minerals, many sicknesses occur. They also feel run-down, cranky, and sick.

Clay assists colon function. Then, the supplements taken in addition to the clay will be better used by the body because it will have the means to do so. The mineral content being high sets the stage for replenishing dietary deficiencies. Today, more than ever before, diets are lacking essential trace minerals and micronutrients. Without the basic minerals, life cannot exist; without trace minerals, major deficiencies may develop. Lack of it will make it impossible for the body to maintain good health and function normally. In clay, the minerals occur in natural proportion to one another encouraging their absorption in the intestinal tract. Natural **Calcium Montmorillonite Clay** restores minerals in the tissues where they are needed. Furthermore, minerals are the carriers of the electrical potential in the cells which enable the hormones, vitamins, and enzymes to function properly.

It is one of the most effective natural intestinal detoxifying agents available and has been recognized as such for centuries by native peoples around the world. Whatever the name, liquid clay contains minerals that, once inside the gastrointestinal tract, are able to absorb toxins and deliver mineral nutrients to an impressive degree, says **Knishinsky**. Liquid clay is inert which means it passes through the body undigested.

Technically, the clay first adsorbs toxins(heavy metals), free radicals, pesticides) attracting them to its extensive surface area where they adhere like flies to sticky paper, then it absorbs the toxins, taking them in the way a sponge mops up a kitchen floor.

Prima, a company based in Ashland, Oregon, which markets Great Plains ® **Bentonite,** the clay's minerals are negatively charged while toxins tend to be positively charged, There is an electrical aspect to bentonite's ability to bind and adsorb toxins. According to **Yerba** hence the clay's attraction works like a magnet drawing metal shavings. But it's even more involved than that.

Once hydrated (combined with water), bentonite has an enormous surface area. According to **Yerba Prima,** a single quart bottle can represent a total surface area of 950 square yards or 12 american football fields. **Bentonite** is made of a great number of tiny platelets, with negative electrical charges on their flat surfaces and positive charges on their edges.

When **bentonite** adsorbs water and swells, it is stretched open like a highly porous sponge; the toxins are drawn into these spaces by electrical attraction and bound fast. In fact, according to the **Canadian Journal of Microbiology (31 (1985),50-53)** bentonite can absorb pathogenic viruses, aflatoxin (a mold) and pesticides and herbicides including Paraquat and Roundup. The clay is eventually eliminated from the body with the toxins bound to its multiple surfaces.

According to **Sonne's Organic Foods** of North Kansas City, Missouri, a company that markets Detoxifant(a liquid montmorillonite), "there is no evidence that bentonite has any chemical action in the body. Its power is purely physical."

Pascalite clay is a calcium bentonite, formed thirty million years ago as the froth and foam of the fiery and convulsive era atop the Big Horn Mountains in Wyoming. It was first used by Indians and for its curative nature and drawing properties, to draw out poisons. **Especially in cases of venomous bites from spiders to snakes. The clay was named Pascalite after a French-Canadian trapper, Emile Pascale.**

The book, "More Precious than Gold" describes many people in Oklahoma being healed of the bite of the brown recluse spider. This spider had caused many deaths and there has been no treatment for it up until recently. In court, one doctor gave evidence of a person being healed by the clay Pascalite of the necrotic wound of the bite of the brown recluse spider.

It is also the only known cure for the bite of the fiddle back spider.

Pascalite clay users have reported many health enhancing results from this wonderful substance. It has been found to have many uses in promoting health in plants, animals and humans. One theory regarding the benefits of Pascalite is that its broad base of minerals serves as an excellent mineral supplement. Technically, Pascalite is a calcium-based, bentonite. Pascalite is believed to not only remove toxins from the body, but also to build up the immune system.

Pascalite is hand mined underground to avoiding contamination, and then solar dried in the high mountains to preserve it's apparent antibiotic qualities. It is then turned into powder to make it readily usable for both internal and well as external usages. Please don't confuse Pascalite with ordinary clays such as bentonite, Jordan Clay or French green clay. Though listed as a calcium bentonite, at least one government agent has hinted it may well be an as-of yet-unidentified material outside the scope of present knowledge.

Dr. Walter Bennet, Ph.D., who investigated it in depth, stated it was a "very mysterious substance".

Clay receives vital energies from sun, air, and waters, making it a powerful agent of stimulation, transformation and transmission of energy.

We all possess energy resources that normally remain dormant. Clay awakens them!

Always make sure that you take clay that meets the stringent U.S federal purity standards for microbial limits, absence of pathogens, and product consistency. Most clays sold in health food stores (in the dietary supplement section) should be safe for consumption.

Make sure the label on the clay you take says "Montmorillonite,"

Not all products on the market can say that NASA has tested them! But Terramin Clay can. Terramin is 100% safe and effective clay that has surpassed all U.S. standards for product purity and consistency. The trade name for pure, high grade edible is Calcium Montmorillonite clay.

Over the centuries, it captured the calcium from that limestone formation, and many other minerals (now known to be vital to life) in trace amounts migrated into it__manganese, cobalt, copper, etc. Technically, Pascalite is a calcium-based bentonite. **Pascalite** is also believed to remove toxins from the body. **Pascalite** is also used as a suppository for **hemorrhoids**. Users found it a potent skin cleanser and conditioner, drank it for heartburn and ulcers. One neglected mineral in **Pascalite**, lately recognized as vital to living tissue, is silica. It is found in Pascalite as silicate and silicones. In the body, silica occurs as collagen, a connective tissue covering the brain, spinal cord, and the nerve systems. It is also an essential part of the hair, skin and nails. Some researchers have hinted that a lack of silica in the brain and nerves may be one cause of poor memory.

It has many other uses. In addition to its other abilities, **Pascalite** has been shown to be an anesthetic. Many users have reported almost immediate cessation of pain following its application in paste form to the areas.

Corns and Calluses:

There have also been testimonies of Pascalite clay being applied on and between the toes for corns and callouses with excellent results.

A wet pack of clay was applied for three days, changed then reapplied for another three days

Chicken Pox:

Add clay to the bath-water to relieve itching which can cause scarring.

Hemorrhoids:

Three individuals stated under oath that topical uses of Pascalite paste had removed all symptoms of hemorrhoids in 2-4 nightly applications. Others reported similar results in use for pile, rectal fissures and related conditions.

In a report by **Dr. Walter W. Bennett, PhD.**, Epistemologist and Research Scientist, who spent several months during 1975 in a very sophisticated examination of **Pascalite**. He reports: *"The presence of protein in this material gives evidence of yet un-disclosed amino acids. The fact that amounts are small, and that even the requirements are for minute quantities in no way diminishes their great importance.*

"Microbiological analysis reveals the interesting fact that the raw material is completely sterile as pertains to any bacteria. However,, it contains the spores of at least 6 different types of fungi.

"When used as a media of raw material it inhibit's the growth of representative pathogens such as staphylococcus, streptococcus, salmonella, Escherichia coli and pseudomonas aerations.

Clay's adsorptive and absorptive qualities may be the key to its multifaceted healing abilities. According to **Knishinsky**, benefits reported by people using liquid clay for a period of two to four weeks include:improved intestinal regularity; relief from chronic constipation, diarrhea, indigestion, and ulcers a surge in physical energy; clearer complexion; brighter, whiter eyes; enhanced alertness; emotional uplift, improved tissue and gum repair; and increased resistance to infections. "Clay works on the entire organism. No part of the body is left untouched by its healing energies.

A medical study by **Frederic Damrau, M.D. in 1961 (Medical Annals of the District of Columbia)** establishes clearly that bentonite can end bouts of diarrhea. When 35 individuals (average age 51) suffering from diarrhea took two tablespoons of bentonite in distilled water daily, the diarrhea was relieved in 97% (34 of the 35 patients) in 3.8 days regardless of the original cause of the problem (allergies, viral infection, spastic colitis, or food poisoning) According to **Dr. Damrau,** bentonite is "safe and highly effective" in treating acute diarrhea.

Knishinsky's research suggests that the regular intake of liquid clay (typically one to three tablespoons daily, in divided doses) can produce other benefits including parasite removal from the intestines, allergy and hay fever relief, and elimination of anemia and acne. For example, clay helps anemia because it contains both types of dietary iron (ferrous and ferric) in an easily assimilated form; it reduces discomfort from allergic reactions, and it reduces heartburn and indigestion by absorbing excess stomach acids.

However, clay's forte is probably its role as a general internal detoxification and cleansing agent. According to **Keith Payne** of **White Rock Mineral Corporation** in **Springville, Utah,** clay scrapes and cleans the lining of the colon. "As the colon becomes cleaner, its ability to adsorb minerals and other nutrients increases, making the minerals even more bioavailability, thus giving more energy.

Bentonite Minerals are derived from an ancient sea bed formation in Utah, according to geologists, the clay formed when a layer of volcanic ash fell into what was,

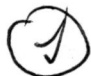

long ago, a shallow inland sea. As the ash filtered through the seawater, it collected pure minerals, forming a layer of highly mineralized clay.

The idea of eating clay to promote internal healing will undoubtedly appear to many as farfetched, if not a little primitive.

However, natural clay, especially in the form known as bentonite, has been used medicinally for hundreds of years by indigenous cultures, and has, in recent years, been increasingly used by practitioners as a simple but effective internal cleanser to help in preventing various health problems.

How do I Take Clay, Internally? Can it be used for children?

The best way to drink clay is on an empty stomach or at least an hour before or after a meal. For best results, Mineral Clay should be taken before going to bed. You can mix it with water or juice. If you find it constipating at first, use prune juice or use a natural laxative until your body becomes regulated. Remember, the clay is "clumping" the toxins together in your body, and is waiting for them to be expelled through the colon... Again, drink plenty of water and natural juices, and exercise in the fresh air. (Also, make sure you are getting a lot of fiber along with the clay.)

Generally, it is advisable to start with one tablespoon daily, mixed with a small amount of juice, observe the results for a week, then gradually increase the dosage to no more than four tablespoons daily, in divided dosages. Drinking clay can be annual spring cleaning of your gastrointestinal tract or it can be symptom-focused, self-care method.

With **children,** you can give ½ teaspoon daily in juice or water.

According to the "**California Wild Magazine**", featuring an article called *Mud Mud, Glorious Mud,* it stated that geophagy (earth-eating) is a well documented phenomenom. In the animal world, parrots seek out particular clays and deer lick hollows into patches of soil, traveling long distances to reach these tasty areas of available soil. Cattle will chew on clods of particular earths; in South Africa, cattle will often be found licking away at termite nests. Termite nests are rich in trace elements, as these "white ants" carry up fragments from as much as a hundred feet down.

Often the ingredient sodium chloride (table salt) is what they are craving, because animals as well as humans need sodium to maintain a proper electrolyte balance, and the chloride ion is a major constituent of stomach acid. Just as often, though, the animals are garnering iron, copper, magnesium, and a host of trace elements up to 65 ingredients, according to South African research work.

If you have animals, you understand that it is necessary to provide them with salt and mineral blocks. Therefore, eating dirt is almost like taking vitamins.

Clay is also an excellent vermifuge, attracting and binding internal parasites and packaging them for disposal.

On the Hawaiian island of Oahu, Kawai Nui Marsh is said to contain a special nutritious mud, called lepo al'ia, and the mud is described in oral traditions recorded by the Bishop Museum in Honolulu as thick and jelly-like the cream color of poi, but with a texture more like pudding. This mud is said to have been specially brought to a fish pond on Kawai Nui by the eleventh century hero, Kaulu-a-Kalana from volcanic pillars off of the coast of the Big Island.

Hawaiian folklore records a siege here around 1795, in King Kamehameha I's time. When the food ran out, Kamehameha ordered his men to eat lepo al'ia. The mud gave the troops enough energy to win the war. Nothing is said of the flavor beyond that it was "pleasing".

The legend's details suggest lepo al'la might well have been a bacterial culture made with mud, just as yogurt is a bacterial culture made with milk. This theory is strengthened by aquatic biologist Eric. B. Guinther's work in Kiribati, an island nation in the South Pacific.

During famines, he writes, the inhabitants survived on a thick gelatinous layer that forms at the bottom of freshwater pits. The mud was dug to grow babai, a taro-like staple food. These slippery masses are especially common in pits on Christmas Atoll. This jelly is a sludge secreted by blue-green algae to protect themselves against extreme salinity .

The cyano bacteria themselves are a relatively small component of the mass, yellow lumps suspended likes cherries in jello.

According to **Guinther,** although this blue-green alga is typically found in highly saline situations, it also occurs in fresh and brackish water, including California reservoirs and the reflecting pool in front of Honolulu's state capital, where it's become an unsightly nuisance. "Whether this is the lep al'ia of Hawaiian legend," he writes, "we simply do not know. But the material would provide some nutrition and would be collected from the bottom mud".

In Peru, the Aymara people of the high Andes have incorporated clays into their daily cuisine. These mountains are the home of the earth-apple, or potato, and the Aymara have thrived for centuries on this reliable food.

It is said that potatoes with even faintly green skins should never be eaten, because of the poisonous glycoalkaloids that develop during germination. Glycoalkaloids can cause diarrhea, vomiting and neurological disturbances, and can be fatal to humans. Many of the half-wild potato species the Aymara eat contain dangerous levels of poison, even before any greening occurs. The aymara cook or steep the tubers with certain kinds of clay to detoxify them. When the clay is drained off, the dish is safe to eat.

The clay adsorbs the glycoalkaloids, allowing toxins to pass harmlessly through the body. Centuries of selective breeding have reduced the amount of poisons produced by the potatoes we eat in the United States. For these potatoes, cooking is sufficient to destroy what little alkaloid remains.

Clay is an essential ingredient in some dishes cooked by indigenous Californians. The Pomo tribe mixes clay with acorn flour to make a bread free of the bitter taste of oak tannins and that is easier to digest. The clay particles stick to the tannin molecules and neutralize them. Because of the very small particle size of clays-as fine as talcum powder-the bread is not gritty.

Pregnant women in many African countries eat white clay to alleviate morning sickness. Anthropologists Boyle and Mackey record the use of clay suspensions in treating nausea in Greece in 40 bc, and it was prescribed by the Roman obstetrician, gynecologist, and pediatrician Soranus of Ephesus, who practiced medicine around 100-140 ad.

Clay, in the form of kaolin, is still a common ingredient in western medicines such as Kaopectate, Rolaids and Maalox. In the stomach, the negative electrical charges of tiny clay particles attract positively charged toxins from stomach fluids. This clumping prevents very tiny particles, such as toxic molecules, from passing through the walls of the intestines and enter the bloodstream.

By clumping together, the poisons pass harmlessly out of the system through the kidneys or bowel. Also, because clays are alkaline, they help neutralize acid poured out by the stomach during digestive disturbances. Once through the stomach and into the intestines, clay particles absorb water and swell. Their presence slows intestinal spasms, easing the symptoms of diarrhea while coating the intestinal walls and protecting against further irritation.

Clay, also helps in early pregnancy when the mother's body is adjusting to the presence and biochemical activity of the fetus. The bland taste of the clay reduces nausea.

As pregnancy advances, the rapidly growing offspring requires large amounts of nutrients, particularly calcium. Without dietary supplements, this calcium can be drawn from the mothers bones. Many women in the past would lose teeth during pregnancy, as calcium withdrawal caused jawbone erosion. Certain clays supply calcium in a form easily used by the body.

Scientific analysis of clays selected by pregnant women

in Nigeria show that eating as little as 500 mg (about the equivalent of two Tylenol capsules) per day can satisfy nearly 80 percent of a pregnant woman's calcium needs. Clay's detoxifying capabilities may also protect the fetus against birth defects that could be caused by plant toxins the mother may eat.

Modern science confirms that minerals derived directly from the earth can be more effective than supplements synthesized by man. In the 1960's when NASA was preparing to conquer space, experiments showed that weightlessness induced

Very rapid bone depletion. Also according to doctors, such conditions weaken the body and increase chances that kidney stones may develop during flights lasting months or years. **Ershoff** found that when tested on animals, that supplementing the diet with calcium alone couldn't reverse the severe damage of severely accelerated osteoporosis; but clay did , for the animals tested. It produced impressive results in promoting growth and preventing disorders in the bones of tested animals.) ***Benjamin Ershoff*** ...They funded a range of pharmaceutical companies to develop calcium supplements. But ***Benjamin Ershoff of the California Polytechnic Institute found that the most efficacious treatment was the tried-and true eating of clay.***

He reported that "the calcium in clay...is adsorbed more efficiently and that it contains some factor or factors other than calcium which promotes improved calcium utilization and / or bone formation." He adds, "Little or no benefit was noted when calcium alone was added to the diet." (When a small amount of the clay was added to the diet, the animals's body weight increased and bone diseases were prevented.)

An article was published on geophogy (clay eating) and detoxification (Timothy and Duquette 1991)

Susanne Ubick is assistant editor of California Wild. (magazine)

According to *Our Earth, Our Cure_Clay Therapy, Healing Clay_Healing Earth*

By Shirley's Wellness Café, Clay is renowned to have many uses in promoting health in plants, animals and humans. Bentonite, Montmorillonite, Pascalite and other types of healing clays, have been used by indigenous cultures since before recorded history. Naturally adsorbent and extreme gentle on the system, bentonite clay can treat various skin and intestinal ailments and attracts and neutralizes poisons in the intestinal tract. It can eliminate food allergies, food poisoning, mucus colitis, spastic colitis, viral infections, stomach flu, and parasites (parasites are unable to reproduce in the presence of clay). There is virtually no digestive disease that clay will not treat. It enriches and balances blood. It adsorbs radiation (cell phones, microwaves, x-rays, color televisions and irradiated foods.

"Russian scientists use bentonite to protect their bodies from radiation when working with nuclear material, by coating their hands and bodies with a hydrated bentonite "magma" before donning radiation suits.) Bentonite adsorbs radiation so well, in fact, that is was the choice material used to dump into Cherynobl after the nuclear meltdown in the former Soviet Union."

During this time in 1986, the Soviet Union put French Green Clay into chocolate bars and dispensed them freely to the masses to remove radiation they may have been exposed to. Found only in France and India, the ancient sea beds that provide the green clays have healing qualities that not only attach themselves to and remove toxic foreign substances within the body, but activate the body's own immune system through its chemical constitution.

Healing Clay and Carpal Tunnel Syndrome:

This article shows how clay can actually relieve the effects of Carpal Tunnel Syndrome.

(Paul R. Martin, McHenry NeuroDiagnostics, McHenry, Illinois, copyright 1996)

Another testimony of a person who stated she was healed of the Carpal Tunnel Syndrome by using clay.

Live2ski@aol.com

Staria L. Allen

In a book by **Wendell Hoffman**, *Using Energy to Heal*, *he found that a special bentonite used in a bath can actually* ***draw out toxic chemical through the pores of the skin.*** After many experiments, he concluded that optimum results are obtained by immersing oneself in a tub of very warm water mixed with bentonite clay for exactly 20 minutes.

Specially formulated clay baths have been shown to be able to literally pull pollutants out like a magnet, getting rid of years of toxic accumulation in just one bath. These clay baths have been scientifically proven to release toxic metals and chemicals from the body, and they are so inexpensive that anyone can afford to take them.

Earth Cures: A Handbook of Natural Medicine for Today by **Raymond Dextreit** states that your cure is not always in the medicine chest, but can be found in your own backyard.....or at your local grocer..This is a valuable book that covers many diseases that clay can assist in healing.

In a wonderful book, **Wild Health:How Animals Keep Themselves Well and What We Can Learn From Them**, By: *Cindy Engles, Ph.D.* devotes an entire chapter to clay -eating). (esophagi) Mammals, birds, reptiles and invertebrates have been observed to eat dirt on every continent except Antartica.

It was even told of ranchers that when their cattle became sick, the animal would actually go off by itself, find some clay and eat it, therefore healing itself. It is said that this practice remains in effect as of today. {*Mahaney, WC Maximilliano, B Hancock, RGV Aufreter, S and Perez, Fl 1996. Geophagy of Holstein hybrid cattle in the northern Andes, Venezuela. Mountain Research and Development, 16(2)pp 177-180.*}

It has been used for alcoholism, arthritis, cataracts, diabetic neuropathy, pain treatment, open wounds, diarrhea, hemorrhoids, stomach ulcers, animal and poisonous insect bites, acne, and anemia. The list goes on. *It was used during the Balkan war of 1910 to reduce mortality **from cholera** among the soldiers from sixty to three percent.*

Again, one has to be totally receptive as to the rewarding benefits of clay . I personally know of people who refuse to receive the what clay has to offer because they look at it as though it is "dirty"; __ this wonderful element that God has given to us.

The native Americans call it "Ee-Wah-Kee" which means "The -Mud_That-Heals".

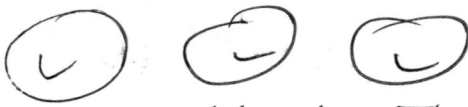

How does This Clay work?

Clay molecules carry a negative electrical charge while impurities carry a positive charge. With the clay the positively charged ions are attracted to the negatively charged surfaces of the clay molecule. An exchange reaction occurs in which the clay mineral ions are swapped for the ions of the positively charged substance. The clay molecule is now electrically satisfied and holds onto the positive ion until our bodies can eliminate both.

Our Earth Our* Cure By *Raymond Dextreit*..**He writes that clay stimulates the deficient organ and help the restoration of the failing function. Clay is a powerful agent of stimulation, transformation and transmission. Clay contains highly active ingredients, able to induce cellular rebuilding and to hasten all organic processes. Used internally, whether adsorbed orally, ***anally or vaginally, clay goes to the place where the problem lies, and there it lodges, until it draws out the infection.....

Note: When mixed with water, clay forms a temporary colloidal system in which fine particles are dispersed throughout the water. Eventually the particles settle to the bottom of the container, but a variety of mineral ions will remain in the water. These mineral ions are available for absorption, while other minerals that form an integral part of the clay particles may, in some circumstances, be available for absorption through ionic exchange at the point of contact with the intestinal villi.

Note: **Ordinary clay can kill the drug-resistant super bug MRSA (methicillin-resistant staphylococcus aureus. *Arizona State University***

Research Dept., also it has been found that some forms of clays actually kill salmonella, E.coli, MRSA

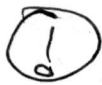

and Mycobacterium ulcerans, which causes flesh-eating disease.

**MRSA is a condition found in many patients in hospitals.

Healing clays have been known for years to soak up toxins produced by bacteria, which can limit the spread of infection. But now, research at Arizona State University shows some forms of clay actually kill salmonella, E.coli, MRSA and Mycobacterium (which causes flesh-eating disease.)

These days, more people are becoming aware of the healing properties in food, herbs, etc. but as of yet, very few know that the earth itself, receiving its vital energies from the sun, air, and waters, is a most powerful healing agent of physical regeneration. Clays, muds, sands---these different forms of earth all participates in life-giving, health restoring processes.

According to ***Jared Diamond*** in an article he wrote on the eating of clay by different birds:

Eat Dirt: in the competition between parrots and fruit trees, it's the winners who bite the dust . **Discover. 19(2) pp70-76**

Adsorption versus Absorbtion:

Adsorbtion:

The two words look alike, but their difference is critical in understanding the functions of clay minerals. **Adsorption** characterizes the process by which

substances stick to the outside surface of the adsorbent medium. The clay possesses unsatisfied ionic bonds around the edges of its mineral particles. It naturally seeks to satisfy those bonds. For this to happen, it must meet with a substance carrying an opposite electrical (ionic) charge. When this occurs, the ions held around the outside structural units of the adsorbent medium and the substance are exchanged.

The particles of clay are said to carry a negative electrical charge, whereas impurities, bacteria, or toxins, carry a positive electrical charge.

The process works the same in the human body. When clay is taken internally, the positively charged toxins are attracted by the negatively charged surfaces of the clay mineral. An exchange reaction occurs whereby the clay exchanges its ions for those of the other substance. Now, electrically satisfied, it holds the toxin in suspension till the body can eliminate both.

The term active, or alive, indicated the ionic exchange capabilities of a given clay mineral. The degree to which the clay-mineral ions become active determine its classification as alive. Living bodies are able to grow and change their form and size by taking within them lifeless material of certain kinds, and by transforming it into a part of themselves. No dead body can adsorb. It is physically impossible.

Absorption:

Absorption is a much more slow and involved process than **adsorption.**

Here, the clay acts more like a sponge, drawing substances into its internal structure. In order for adsorption to occur, the substance must undergo a chemical change to penetrate the medium's barrier. Once it has done that, it enters between the unit layers of the structure. Instead of the toxins, for instance, sticking only to the surface, they are actually pulled inside the clay. This is the reason why absorptive clays are labeled expandable clays. The more substances the clay absorbs into its internal structure, the more it expands and its layers swell.

Any clay mineral with an inner layer charge is an absorbent. Having an inner layer charge means having charged ions, sitting between layers, that are surrounded by water molecules. In this way, the clay will expand as the substance to be absorbed fills the spaces between the stacked silicate layers.

Some clays are more gentle in their absorption, whereas others are definetly more radical. Absorption takes place with clay when the clay draws particulates into its internals layered structure, much like a sponge. Clay minerals have an inner layer charge that acts like an adsorbent and can absorb and bond with many elements that are toxic, both man-made and natural.

The smaller the particle size of clay, the more platelets there are per given cubic centimeter of volume or unit of weight and the larger the total surface area is. Their **absorbent** and **adsorbent** capacity increases with the numbers of clay platelets per given unit of measure. The natural parent size of clay particles are created by nature is fixed. The industrial process of crushing, grinding, milling, etc. will not change the parent particle size once created. They do clump or bond together many times making them larger in size, however processing it mechanically can make them no smaller than nature originally created.

Clays are like people, there are no two alike. Each clay deposit on earth has its own type. This unique identity is

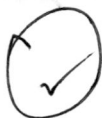

comprised of it particular composition of the elements on the periodic table, different ratios to one another, differed ionic electrical charge, different particle size, different purity, different exposure for a different amount of time, to mention a few of the differences. As a result of some of these differences, they react accordingly different when applied or utilized. Some clays "work" while others do not, or not very well for the intended purpose.

I would advise one to experiment with the different clays to find what is good for oneself.

I have listed many references in the back of this book.

Examples of other purposes that the beneficial effects clay provides are:

Aquaculture :

Ponds and Waterways

(Clay added to the water results in healthy Koi fish.) It helps by eliminating waste products, bacteria and decomposed organic matter in the water. When these particles are absorbed safely, it will result in healthy fish and clear, clean pond water.

Clay can also be added to aquariums to control the growth of algae.

Note:
The benefits of clay mentioned in this book have only touched the surface of The Healing Essentials of Clay.

As there are no dangers to fear using clay(there is no reason to oppose giving it a try.)

I also thank all of the individuals who have contributed to the benefits of clay research.

Bibliography

Check your local library and online for more information about healing clays.

U.S. Geological Survey

Hosterman, J.W. and Patterson, S.H. 1992 Bentonite and fuller's earth resources of the United States: U.S. Geological Survey Bulletin 1522, 45 p

Papke, Keith G., 1970, Montmorillonite, Bentite, and fuller's earth deposits in Nevada

14-16, 1974: Georgia Department of Natural Resources, Guidebook 14, 53 p.
Robertson, R.H.S, 1986. Fuller's earth-a history of calcium and montmorillonite: Volturna Press, Hythe, UK, no. 18, 421 p.

Knishinsky, Ran. The Clay Cure

Honey, Mud, Maggots and Other Medical Marvels by Robert and Michele Root-Bernstein

Jensen, Neva. The Healing Power of Living Clay

Walter Wilett. Eat, Drink and be Healthy

Geffen, David. Guns, Germs and Steel

Engles, Cindy, Ph.D. Wild Health: How animals

keep themselves well and what we can learn from them

Dextreit, Raymond . Earth Cures . A Handbook of Natural Medicine for today

Hay, Louise . You can Heal Yourself

Levine, Barbara . Your Body Believes Every Word You Say

Payne, Keith . White Rock Mineral Corp, Springville, Utah

Ershoff, Benjamin . California Polytechnic Institute

Price, Dr. Weston A. DDS. Nutrition and degeneration. Keats Publishing .1939

Live2ski2@AOL.com (carpal tunnel syndrome recovery testimony)
Staria L. Allen

Clay Distributors:

Red Desert Clay
Maryanne Maldonado (Wellness Coach) (clay
distributor and lecturer)
520-219-2379

Shirley's Wellness Café (clay distributor)
Shirley Lipschultz Robinson (natural Wellness
Researcher)
206-984-3009 or
323-389-0560
Laura Curtiss @ 713-408-1707 (Natural Health
Mentor, Consultant and Clay

Lauana Lei's Magnetic Clay Baths
LL's Magnetic Clay, Inc.
800-257-3315
Contact: Judy Phillips, owner

Uncle Harry's Natural Products
425-558-4251
Clay Distributor

Sales@specialclay.com
Pascalite clay distributor

Pascalite, Inc.
307.347.2346 (fax)
307.347.3872 (phone)
Distributor

Dead Sea Products
Bath salts, etc. (External Mineral Mud from the Dead
Sea for face and body)
Cleopatra' Choice
1-800-925-4232
(They will furnish a certificate of authenticity
Contact:Sharon Allen

Clay Has Been Known To Benefit These Ailments:

Osteoporosis
Cancer
Gout
Sty(Inflammation of the eyelid)
Carpal Tunnel Syndrome
Psoriasis (various skin ailments, acne, etc.)
Cuts (Abrasions)
Hair growth
Scalp disorders, etc. (dandruff)
Foot disorders (sprains, etc)
Yeast infections (vaginal problems)
Rectal problems (hemorrhoids, fissures, etc.)
Tooth infection
Pyorrhea(gum disease)
Poison ivy, poison sumac
Digestion(there is virtually no digestive disease that clay
will not treat.)
Circulation Problems
Menstruation
Liver Problems
Prostate
Arthritis
Chronic Fatigue Syndrome
Gum Disease (pyorrhea)
Migraines
Ganglion and sub-aceous cycts and Boils
Chicken Pox (itching relief)
Corns, Callouses
Insect Stings (spider bites, brown recluse and fiddle

spider)
Animal (pet illnesses)
diarrhea
Diabetic neuropathy
Pain treatment
Swelling(edema)
Enrichment and balance of blood
Parasites
Cholera
Radiation adsorption
Cataracts

(The list is too long for this book.)

This is a book exploring the many benefits of the Healing Essentials of Clay.

Therefore we do not lost heart, though outwardly we are wasting away, yet inwardly we are being renewed day by day. For our light and momentary troubles are achieving for us in eternal glory that far outweighs them all. So we fix our eyes not on what is seen, but on what is unseen. For what is seen is temporary, but what is unseen is eternal.

2 Corinthians 4:16-18